The Two-Week
Wellness Solution

The Two-Week Wellness Solution

The Fast Track to Permanent Weight Loss and Vitality!

Tess Challis

Published by Quintessential Health Publishing
P.O. Box 1784
Pagosa Springs, CO 81147
www.RadiantHealth-InnerWealth.com

Printed in the United States of America
First edition 2010

Cover photographs of the author by Jeff Laydon

Food photographs on the cover (left to right):
Ever So Nice Beans and Rice (by Olga Vasiljeva), *Rawberry Star Bars* (by Olga Vasiljeva), *Apricot-Glazed Asparagus* (by Olga Vasiljeva), *Sunshine Smoothie* (by Olga Vasiljeva), and *Spinach Strawberry Salad* (by Michelle McCluggage). Photo on the spine of *Holiday Waffles* by Michelle McCluggage.

ISBN# 1452851867

This book is dedicated to you.
May you align with your highest state of wellness
and live a joyful, fulfilled life.

In Gratitude
· · · · · · · · · · ·

As with any creative project, this book is the result of many wonderful people being wonderful. First of all, I feel such gratitude towards my mother, Kathryn Barnes. Her passion for organic gardening inspired me at a young age, and she was the first one to teach me how to prepare whole foods with love.

Thanks also to my uncle, Mark Challis, for being an inspiring role model for life-long vegetarianism and great health. My grandma, Patricia Challis, also deserves many thanks for helping me through college, where I first began to study holistic health and nutrition.

Sheila Barrows, a brilliant editor, is owed an incredible debt of gratitude for her patience, generosity, and great advice. What would I have done without her? Seriously, it wouldn't have been pretty.

Many thanks also to the fabulous Lisa Bagchi for reading through the book and giving me her valuable feedback. Thanks also to Jennifer Sawyer-Byrne, Stacey Groth, and Natalie Carpenter for their helpful, enthusiastic advice and assistance.

I also owe many thanks to all of the wonderful recipe testers. Because of their feedback, each recipe is better than it would have been without their input. Many thanks to Jeananne Libbert, Erica Hunter, Jennie Blechman, Tracy Riley, Stacey Groth, Sherrie Thompson, Monica Valencia, Laura Amber-O'Sullivan, Laura Daniels, Amy Silver, Mary-Allison Hall, and Nancy Mosher. Thank you so much!

Many thanks also go to Jennie Blechman, who was the first person to stick with this program for the whole two weeks. She confirmed everything I'd hoped about this plan, which inspired me share it with others who would also benefit.

I feel infinite gratitude toward the group of women who generously shared their success stories in this book. Thanks to Erica Hunter, Danielle Schmidt, Jennie Blechman, Alison Ronn, Millisa Barron Davis, Rebecca A. Weaver-Gill, Sarah Wright, Laura Amber-O'Sullivan, Rosine Stout, Shonna Lovett Mackelprang, Tracy Riley, Sherrie Thompson, Mary-Allison Hall, Bobbie Rapp, and Tami Kowal. You are all my heroes!

Thanks also to Jeff Laydon for being such a wonderful photographer. He actually turned my dread of doing a photo shoot into a really fun day! Hyla Molander also deserves many thanks for her assistance with the photographs—such a talented photographer (and writer)!

My daughter, Alethea, also gets a big fat thank you for all of the hours she put up with her mom working incessantly while she had to keep herself entertained! It was a lot to ask of a six-year-old (now seven), but she was an angel.

I would also like to thank Bulleh Shah for his endless support on every level. There is no way this book would have happened without him.

Many thanks to Jill Eckart for her diligence, enthusiasm, and kindness. I am also most appreciative of Dr. Neal Barnard and Robert Cheeke—despite their hectic schedules, they made the time to review the book of a little-known author. I will never forget that kindness.

Olga Vasiljeva is due a debt of gratitude for once again enthusiastically taking such beautiful food photographs. Such talent! Michelle McCluggage also deserves many thanks for taking such gorgeous food photographs for me. Thanks so much, beautiful ladies!

Finally, I feel so grateful for all the encouragement my students and clients have given me over the years. Your support has always meant more to me than you could ever know. Without you, I would have never kept going.

Thanks so much. You are all deeply, deeply appreciated!

Foreword

· · · · · · ·

In **The Two-Week Wellness Solution**, you'll get the green light to, as Tess says, "love the foods that love you back." Tess's plan gets you on the path to great health on the inside and out!

Our research at the Physicians Committee for Responsible Medicine has shown that switching to a plant-based diet brings so many benefits: renewed energy, a youthful heart, and much less risk for the illnesses that affect so many people. In fact, our research shows that a vegan diet can reverse type 2 diabetes, tackle cholesterol problems, and conquer long-standing weight challenges.

This book provides you with the total health package—inspiring success stories, frequently asked questions, grocery lists, and a step-by-step plan to get you feeling great and losing weight within no time at all. And the recipes are dynamite! You don't have to read further than the name of the recipe: "Veggie Vitality Juice," "Apple Pie Amaranth Oatmeal," "Spicy Sweet Potato Fries," and "In a Hurry? Curry!" to want to leap into your kitchen and start the process.

Neal Barnard, M.D., President
Physicians Committee for Responsible Medicine

Contents

· · · · · ·

Author's Note
· · · · · · · · · · · ·

Are you wondering what makes this book, this plan, different from all the other weight loss programs? That's a great question! First of all, this program functions as a cleanse—as a way to detoxify from all the bad habits and unhealthy foods we've subjected our bodies to over the years. However, unlike most other detoxification plans, this program doesn't involve going hungry or depriving yourself of tasty food. The one thing I hear constantly from the participants is that they never felt hungry during the two weeks. And they always tell me how great they feel while on the program and how much they love the food.

Another aspect that sets the Two-Week Wellness Solution apart is that it really works. Not only do the participants gain a plethora of health benefits, they also lose weight—usually more than they ever thought possible—during the two weeks. And they keep it off. This is because they love the food and health benefits so much that they don't want to go back to their unhealthy habits.

However, what's really exciting to me is that this isn't just about weight loss. It's about *healthy* weight loss. Sustainable weight loss. The last thing I'd ever want to do is create yet another gimmick for quick weight loss at the expense of health and wellness. No. That has already been done far too often. Instead, this plan will help you to become healthy quickly and stay healthy for the rest of your life.

The idea is to use the two weeks to jump-start your weight loss, detoxify your body, and learn some healthy new habits that you can enjoy maintaining for life. You will learn to make foods that taste fantastic and, at the same time, nourish you and support your well-being. With this program, you will experience a greater wellness—both inner and outer—that will become a new way of being for you. You will gain energy, correct existing health problems, and feel lighter and better than ever.

Which brings me to a point. I believe that, although this program will help you to lose weight quickly, it's meant to bring you to your healthiest weight. It's meant to make you fit and healthy for life. Especially for women, this is a very important point to understand. We have been inundated for decades with images of stick-thin models, and we have judged our own bodies as compared to them. However, I'd like to suggest a new standard to live by—that **healthy is beautiful**. When you use this two-week program to gain health and lose weight, I'd like to encourage you to love yourself and your body as much as you can in the process. Don't try to be too thin or fit into a size zero. There's enough of that craziness in the world already. I'd like to suggest that you eat for health (which this plan will teach you to do), eat enough, listen to your body, be happy, and enjoy life. See how beautiful and lovable you already are and use this program to become even more healthy and happy! Best wishes for your success in every way.

With Love,

Introduction

· · · · · · · · · ·

Do you believe that you have to suffer in order to have the body you want? Do you think it's necessary to endure rigid fasting practices in order to detoxify your body? Have you been caught in the diet trap for most of your life, counting calories and depriving yourself? If your answer to any of these questions is yes, then you're in for a pleasant surprise. You are about to discover a whole new way of eating—one that will simultaneously satisfy your taste buds and allow you to become your healthiest, most radiant self. My motto is "Thrive, don't deprive!" The Two-Week Wellness Solution will help you meet your weight loss goals in record time (most of my participants lose a full dress size in just two weeks!). However, more importantly, it will teach you how to enjoy truly health-giving foods—foods that nourish and support your wellness and ensure that you'll live a long and healthy life.

So, how exactly is this plan different from all of the other diets out there? First of all, it's not a "diet." It's a whole new way of eating. And while many other programs work in the short term, few provide a really healthy long-term solution. After losing some weight, the participants usually go back to their old habits, often regaining even more weight and feeling guilty about their "failure." However, I'm here to tell you (and I want you to really hear this): It's not your fault! You were probably well intentioned, but you were following a plan that wasn't truly supportive to you in the long run.

On the other hand, the program in this book has been designed for maximum short-term success as well as long-term maintainability. In other words, the first two weeks will substantially kick-start your weight loss goals and detoxify your body—but that's just the beginning. After the two weeks, you can continue the plan as is, or follow one of the even more flexible "after-plans" (pages 187-191). This will ensure that you find a custom fit for your eating personality, which will in turn keep you naturally fit and healthy for life.

In a nutshell, this program will help you to lose weight, detoxify and cleanse your system, lower your cholesterol, improve your mood, increase your energy, boost your immune function, and look and feel your absolute best—all while enjoying delicious foods at every meal and never having to go hungry! On the whole, this is a plan for people like me—I love food (a little too much, admittedly), but I don't want what I eat to keep me from experiencing my highest level of health. By developing this plan (and lots of delicious recipes), my message is that you **can** have it all—both the satisfaction of enjoying every bite of food you eat, as well as the joy and peace that comes with a truly healthy body.

It's also important to note that no matter what you've done up until this point, you really can make powerful, positive changes. No matter how much weight you want to lose or how poor your health has become, you can begin right now to turn things around and become that shining, radiantly healthy version of yourself. The human body is an amazing thing, designed to be fit and healthy. When we eat the right foods, our bodies naturally and effortlessly function in a state of complete wellness. However, too many people today have forgotten this and have come to regard disease and health problems as a normal part of life. This plan will restore your natural state of total wellness by removing the things that get in the way, such as refined flours, animal products, hydrogenated oils, and artificial ingredients. Uh-oh—wait a minute! Were those the main things you were eating before? Were you living on fast food or frozen dinners? Does the thought of a healthy vegan diet send up red flags that say "Put this book down and run to the nearest donut store?" Please relax. Let me tell you a story.

One of the participants in this program was eating that way before she started the two-week plan. In fact, she said a typical day for her included a big breakfast, pizza for lunch, fast food on the way home from work (a hamburger and a fish sandwich, along with a shake and some fries), and then a big dinner. However, when she really took the time to pay attention, she began to realize that she had actually stopped enjoying those foods. Although the thought of switching to a vegan diet was frightening to her, she finally decided to try it for the two weeks. To her absolute surprise, she not only lost lots of weight and experienced countless health benefits, but she also began to enjoy food again for the first time in years! The new flavors were so appealing to her and she finally, finally felt satisfied after eating. I still remember the day she e-mailed me to say she was full after eating some miso soup and a salad for lunch. This was significantly lower in calories than what she had been eating, but yet she felt full!

In fact, I've heard this from many others as well. This is because the foods on this program are so high in nutrients that the participants finally began to get clear "I'm full" signals from their bodies. Previously, their bodies were too confused—

although they were getting more than enough calories, the foods the participants had been eating had very little nutritional value. So they just kept eating and eating, subconsciously trying to nourish their bodies with nutrient-poor foods. However, when people begin to eat healthy, plant-based foods, their bodies automatically know when they've eaten enough. This is, in fact, one of the main reasons there is no need to count calories on this program.

So, as I would with anything else, I ask you to approach this plan with an open mind. Don't tell yourself you're going to be a health-food vegan for the rest of your life (unless you really feel you can). Just try it for the two weeks. Chances are, you'll soon begin to wonder why you'd ever want to eat anything else. Your health will improve, you'll begin to look and feel incredible, and you'll develop a whole new repertoire of delectable comfort foods that won't slow you down or compromise your health.

And remember—a healthy vegan diet isn't about what you're missing. It's about what you're gaining. Not only will it provide you with a fit, trim, healthy body for life (and allow you to live longer in that ideal body!), it will also ease your conscience—a vegan diet is much more humane to animals as well as easy on our increasingly fragile ecosystem. Plus, once you get the hang of cooking up fabulous plant-based cuisine, your tastes will change dramatically. You will find animal-based foods and other unhealthy choices to be distasteful. You will eventually even stop craving them completely—believe me.

So, my final advice? Just try it. What do you have to lose (other than excess weight, high cholesterol, and premature aging)? Most importantly, ask yourself what you have to gain. Wouldn't it be wonderful if you really could achieve all of your health goals, learn to love foods that always love you back, and live a long, remarkably healthy life? The good news is that you can! And you can begin right now. I wish you much success and happiness on your journey!

The Two-Week Wellness Solution

· ·

In this chapter, you'll find out what the Two-Week Wellness Solution is all about and why it will transform your health, body, and mood. So, sit down and put your feet up—your life is about to get really good!

The Two-Week Wellness Solution: An Overview

In a nutshell, this plan is about eating delicious, low-fat, plant-based whole foods. To make things as simple and straightforward as possible, I've also color-coded my recipes to help you make great choices. "Green" recipes are to be emphasized—they're light, low in fat, and high in fiber. "Blue" recipes are also acceptable, but in moderation. Although they're essentially healthy, they often include higher-fat plant foods or natural sweeteners. As a guideline, up to one serving of a "blue" recipe daily is fine on this program. The only other "rules" (and I use that term loosely) are that you drink plenty of water, eat six servings of vegetables daily, begin an exercise routine, get some fresh air daily, don't overeat, and take your best shot at the inner wellness basics (pages 20-23).

Although that sounds simple enough, I realize that for many of you it might seem overwhelming. However, many of my most successful clients lived on fast food, never exercised, and hated vegetables before they started this program. And I know without a doubt that if they can do it, so can you. In the "Two-Week Rock Stars" chapter, you'll read about Danielle, a woman who made just such a drastic change. However, she knew her health was too important to put off caring for it any longer and really committed herself to the program. In just three weeks, she lost 25 pounds! And, even more exciting, she's still thriving and loving her new lifestyle today. So, take heart. No matter what you were doing up until this point, know that you can transform your life, your habits, and your body. And you can make it a fun, permanent change!

Finally, remember that the basic program is only two weeks long. You can do anything for just two weeks, right? After the two weeks are up, you can evaluate your progress and decide where you want to go with it from there.

Why The Two-Week Wellness Solution is Your Solution

Chances are, you've tried other diets. You've experimented with all kinds of weight loss plans. You've either gone on fasts and cleanses before, or you've thought about doing so. However, you've come right back to the place you are now—you know your health needs improvement, but you haven't found a way to make positive changes stick. You feel frustrated in your attempts to achieve lasting health and wellness and have even felt like giving up at times. Plus, if you're anything like me, you like food a little too much. You don't want to suffer through weeks (heck, even days) of deprivation.

First things first—give yourself a hug. Know that you're not alone. Because I'll tell you, the longer I live (and work as a wellness coach), the more I see that almost everyone has gone through dieting extremes. Even people we see as supremely healthy have all had their battles. Most of us have also alternated between extremes far too often—we say "I can't eat that" and deprive ourselves, but we end up overeating half the time! Can you relate? I know I can! I spent almost all of my twenties as an obese vegan (yes, it's possible) because I was caught up in dieting extremes. It wasn't until I learned to find balance that I stopped overeating, started listening to my body, and actually learned how to truly enjoy food again—without the guilt! Because enjoying food is part of what will help you regain balance and once again restore your body to a state of perfect health.

So, food lovers, rest easy! With the Two-Week Wellness Solution, you'll learn how to love foods that actually love you back. By making healthy foods that taste amazingly good, you'll retune your taste buds and body and quickly stop craving junk. Plus, you'll only eat when you're hungry, which will ensure that you'll actually enjoy your food more. Remember, my motto is "Thrive, don't deprive!"

Simply put, the enjoyment factor is one of the main reasons why this program will work for you and has worked for so many others—it puts an end to deprivation, guilt, and dieting extremes. It cleanses your body without fasting or arduous detoxification. It ensures that you will lose weight quickly, but without the annoyance of counting calories or putting your olives on a scale before you eat. This plan will work for you because it's about a real solution. A solution that involves listening to your body, giving it the foods it craves, and letting yourself enjoy one of life's simple pleasures—eating. When the two weeks are up, every participant I've ever worked with has told me that they wanted to stick with the program. This is because they loved the food and didn't want to give up all of the benefits they'd gained by following this plan. They had a new lease on life that felt rewarding and exciting. If you choose to complete this program, you too will be empowered, happy, and healthy—and you'll have a whole new repertoire of delicious foods that will keep you fit and satisfied. And trust me, you deserve it!

How The Two-Week Wellness Solution Works

This program works in a very natural, intuitive way by combining structure with freedom. In my experience, that concept alone is key. Too much structure makes us want to rebel and go crazy on chocolate bunnies, while too much freedom can make us feel unsupported. This program works so well because it keeps you in check while simultaneously letting you do some customizing. You can literally have your cake and eat it too on this plan—and know that the cake won't leave you with regrets (for once)!

Here are the key points of this program and some of their benefits:

• Each morning, you'll start your day off with fresh lemon water. This will wake up your system with a gentle liver detoxification. Plus, lemon water is perfect for helping to cleanse and alkalinize your body, as well as being immune-boosting and highly nutritive.

• Next, you'll continue to break your nightly fast (the time between your evening meal and breakfast) with fruit. This gently works with our systems, not against them, as our bodies digest fruit quickly and easily.

• After you've given your lemon water and fruit a little time to digest, you'll begin to eat foods that require more from your digestive system. However, at this point your body has been cleansed, is hungry, and can easily take on more complex foods. You can consume any "green" foods (foods in this book labeled as "green") mid-morning, and they'll keep you going until lunch.

• At lunchtime, you'll start off with two cups of vegetables. Fresh vegetables contain loads of beneficial enzymes that stimulate and greatly aid your digestive process. Also, as you'll be prioritizing your vegetable intake by eating them first, you're sure to fill up without consuming too many calories. You'll also be guaranteed plenty of fiber, vitamins, and nutrients. Of course, if you're eating an entrée that already contains two cups of vegetables (such as the "Garlic Veggie Noodle Bowl, Your Way"), you can skip the step of eating your vegetables first and instead enjoy them as the primary part of your meal. Any "green" foods are fine for lunchtime, in addition to your happy veggies.

• You'll eat another meal at around 3 p.m., which will also consist of the two cups of vegetables and "green" foods. This mid-afternoon meal is essential, as it will ensure that you don't overeat at dinner—plus, you'll keep your metabolism going strong by never allowing yourself to get too hungry.

• At 3 p.m. you'll also stop eating starches for the rest of the day. After this time, you'll only be consuming vegetables and beans. Although this sounds strict, there are still lots of delicious foods you can eat (see p. 16 for dinner ideas). The reason for this is to greatly speed up cleansing and weight loss during the two weeks. Originally a fitness trainer "trick," this cutoff time ensures that you're consuming a minimum of calories in the evenings. When your metabolism is at its slowest, you won't have all kinds of extra calories (from pastas, etc.) to burn off. This will also give your system longer to cleanse each day, as you won't have a big meal to digest. And remember, you can always add healthy starches (complex carbohydrates) back into your evening meal once you've detoxified using the two-week plan.

• You'll be drinking three quarts (or more) of water each day, which will keep your skin glowing, your system cleansing, and your, uh, bowels moving. A little too much information perhaps, but true. Additionally, the body's signals for thirst can often feel like hunger signals. Staying well hydrated will ensure that you're only eating when you're truly hungry—not just thirsty.

• You will not be consuming fiber-free animal products or refined foods during this plan, so you'll keep your system clean and functioning at its peak. High-fiber foods are a key to weight loss and overall health—plus, fiber-rich foods keep you full much longer and therefore assist you in consuming less food in general.

• For those of you who feel your bodies need to detoxify, you're in for a treat! You'll be thoroughly cleansed on this plan, but without having to undergo the stress of rigorous fasting. Plus, at the end of the two weeks, you'll actually know how to live a healthy lifestyle—versus a typical fast or cleanse where you never really learn how to eat right long-term.

• Consuming plenty of water and vegetables, listening to your body (and not overeating), and emphasizing high-fiber "green" foods will eliminate any need for counting calories. You'll automatically consume the right amount of calories to lose weight just by doing these simple things. The human body is truly amazing. It will function at optimum levels with ease—all we have to do is get out of the way and let it!

• Emphasizing recipes with the "green" label (with up to one serving of a "blue"-labeled recipe daily) will keep your fat and sugar consumption in check, while still allowing you to enjoy tasty foods. Again, no calorie counting!

• You're also encouraged to begin an exercise routine during the two weeks. Ideally, 30 minutes or more of exercise daily is a great goal. However, as everyone's fitness levels vary, my advice is to start with a doable foundation of exercise that you can continue to build on for the rest of your life.

• I recommend spending at least ten minutes outside each day (although more is even better, of course). This will elevate your mood and increase your vitamin D levels naturally.

• The "Inner Wellness Basics" (pages 20-23) are also recommended for the two-week plan. They'll boost your energy levels, help you reach your goals quickly and easily, and get you in touch with your wise inner self.

• You'll also be asked to listen to your body and pay attention to your level of hunger and fullness (as explained on p. 12). This alone will assist you greatly in achieving your weight loss goals, as only you know what your body is saying at any given time. The best thing you can do is to become your own best expert on your body and give it exactly what it needs, in exactly the right amounts.

The Hunger and Fullness Gauge

This is a guideline that you can refer to throughout the day and while you're eating. With practice, it will help you become your own best nutritionist! Simply listening to your body and giving it the right amount of food will go a long, long way in helping you maintain your ideal weight for life. Although it takes practice to listen to your body, it will become second nature over time.

Here are the different levels of hunger and fullness:

1. You're so hungry that you feel ravenous! You might have trouble concentrating and you may even feel weak. Headaches, stomach pains, crankiness, and dizziness are also possible at this level because of excessive hunger. If you allow yourself to get to this point, you will be much more likely to make unconscious choices about what you eat, as well as how much to eat. You are just too darn hungry to think straight!

2. You're hungry, but aren't experiencing the negative side effects of the first level.

3. You have eaten *just* enough to satisfy your hunger. Your taste buds and habits may entice you to eat more, but your body would feel fine without more food. You feel light, nourished, and physically satisfied. Try to gravitate toward this ideal level as much as you possibly can.

4. You have eaten past the point of simply satisfying your physical hunger. You still feel fine for the most part, but are a little full. You didn't need to eat quite as much as you did.

5. You have eaten so much that you feel very unpleasantly full. You may have binged, or you may have even started eating when you weren't hungry. Any eating at this stage is a form of self-sabotage and abuse. However, you can heal this habit, no matter how long you have been in this cycle!

One way to begin using this gauge is to simply check in with your body several times a day. Each time, try to identify which level you're at. Next, become very familiar with how you feel, physically and emotionally, at each level you find yourself at. You may find it particularly helpful to pay special attention to how you feel at level three. Try to bring more awareness to that healthy place, as what we focus on is what expands. If we focus on where we do want to be (instead of where we don't want to be), we will find ourselves there more and more consistently!

What this Program Will Do For You

After working with dozens of participants on this program, I can honestly say that the Two-Week Wellness Solution can make miracles happen! People have reported everything from major drops in cholesterol and weight to a remarkable improvement in their mood and complexion. And although everyone is different and there are no 100 percent guarantees, you should experience these benefits too if you're faithful to the program and stick with it. I want **you** to be a rock star in my next book!

The following are examples of what you can expect, based on what I repeatedly hear from participants of this program:

• Your system will cleanse and detoxify naturally without fasting or deprivation.

• You will drop weight quickly and safely.

• You will get strong, lean, and fit—no matter what your age.

• Your complexion will glow and radiate health.

• Your cholesterol will decrease (and if you stick with the plan, it will soon stabilize at your ideal level).

• You will learn to distinguish between true and false cravings (what your body really needs and wants versus what your taste buds are hankering for).

• The program will give you renewed hope and an exciting new lease on life.

• You will experience greater and greater levels of joy, gratitude, well-being, and peace.

• You will no longer feel bloated or be constipated—you'll be as regular as a sunrise (or sunset, whichever you prefer).

• For women (and let's face it, sister—most of you reading this are) who are still menstruating, you'll be very pleased with how much easier your life will get in that area. Your cramps will diminish, your flow will be reduced, and your PMS will be going, going, gone!

• You will have all kinds of energy! No more afternoon drop or evening crash. You'll enjoy consistent energy throughout each day.

• Your immune system will function at a far higher level—it will be much harder to catch illnesses, and if you do, they will be milder and shorter in duration.

• Your risk for heart disease, cancer, and other life-threatening illnesses will be greatly reduced by eating a healthy vegan diet. Plus, you'll most likely live longer—and enjoy excellent health at every stage of your life.

• You'll soon prefer this new way of eating. You'll discover a whole new world of delicious foods that your whole family will love. Foods that don't nourish your body will become distasteful to you, and you'll completely stop craving junk.

• You will learn to listen to your body and give it exactly what it needs at all times.

A Day in the Life of the Two-Week Plan

Here's what a typical day looks like on the program. Keep in mind that there's a complete two-week menu and shopping guide (pages 63-78) if you'd rather have someone else (me) do your meal planning for you. Also take into account that you can eat up to one serving of a "blue" food each day (as long as it's not after the 3 p.m. meal).

Morning:

First thing: Lemon Water (see p. 84 for more details)
Optional: 1-2 tablespoons "Green Radiance" (p. 86) mixed with water
Next: 1-2 servings of fresh fruit (or a fruit smoothie)

Mid-morning (optional, if you're hungry): A "green" snack

Examples (choose one of the following):

High-fiber breakfast cereal with nondairy milk
2-3 "Rawsome Energy Cookies" (p. 134)
Two fresh spring rolls (if you're kooky like me)

Lunch:

First thing: Two cups of vegetables (the fresher the better)
Second thing: Any "green" foods (Don't eat past level three on the hunger and fullness gauge, located on p. 12.)

3 p.m. mini-meal:

First thing: Two cups of vegetables (the fresher the better)
Second thing: Any "green" foods (Don't eat past level three on the hunger and fullness gauge.)

After the 3 p.m. mini-meal:

You will only be consuming beans and vegetables after this cutoff time. It's also best to keep your total fat intake under two teaspoons after 3 p.m.

Dinner:

First thing: Two cups of vegetables (the fresher the better)
Any of the "green" bean dishes or soups (Don't eat past level three on the hunger and fullness gauge.)

Note: Many people find that a salad and soup make a nice evening meal on this program.

Examples of evening entrées from the recipes in this book:

- Ful Mudhamas (p. 57)
- Perfect Pinto Beans (p. 109)
- Black-eyed Peas with Kale (p. 162)
- Five-Minute Five-Bean Salad (p. 115)
- Get Skinny Soup (p. 146)
- Hearty Vegetarian Chili (p. 152)
- Mediterranean Chickpea Salad (p. 113)
- In a Hurry? Curry! (p. 160)
- Moroccan French Lentils (p. 163)
- Simply Soothing Fresh Tomato Soup (p. 148)
- Savory Sage and Red Lentil Soup (p. 149)
- Lickety Split Pea Soup (p. 147)
- Garam Masala Chickpea Curry (p. 168)

Additional ideas for entrées from *Radiant Health, Inner Wealth*:

- Yummy Fat-Free Refried Beans
- Moong Dal
- Easy Indian Mung Beans
- Rosemary White Beans with Artichokes and Sun-Dried Tomatoes
- Light Night Asparagus-Bean Curry
- Fat-Free Red Lentils & Spinach with Tamarind
- Red Lentil, Spinach, & Lemon Soup
- Lemon-Ginger Miso Medicine
- Immune Power Soup

Overall requirements to be filled throughout the day:

• 3-4 quarts of fresh, filtered (or spring) water (If you like, you can add lemon juice or "Green Radiance" to your water or substitute non-caffeinated herbal tea.)

• The vegetable requirement each day is a total of six cups—and at least four cups of the vegetables should be eaten raw and uncooked.

• At least ten minutes of being outside in the fresh air

• This is a great time to begin an exercise program (after consulting with your health care practitioner). Aim for at least 30 minutes of exercise daily as your goal, but keep it doable.

Inner Wellness Basics (see pages 20-23 for details):

• Look in the mirror once each day and say "I love myself" (and/or "I am open to loving myself more").

• Think of at least five things you are grateful for each morning or evening.

• Visualize being the ideal version of yourself.

• Meditate for at least five minutes (or just sit quietly and observe your thoughts).

Two-Week Do's

The following foods are great choices for the two-week plan:

• Whole foods (foods that are in their whole, natural state) such as vegetables, potatoes, yams, brown rice, amaranth, quinoa, beans, legumes, and fruits get my enthusiastic thumbs up during this plan! They are nourishing, low-fat, high-fiber foods that help our bodies thrive.

• Tempeh, when prepared with a minimum of oil, is an excellent choice. For those unfamiliar with this uber-nutritious fermented food, tempeh is delicious in all kinds of things—sloppy joes, fajitas, sandwiches, wraps, and Mexican dishes. Just make sure to marinate your tempeh before cooking it, as it will have much more flavor that way!

• For more ideas, see the acceptable "green" packaged foods listed on pages 181-185.

These foods are acceptable in moderation during the two weeks:

• Higher-fat plant foods (avocado, nuts, seeds, nut and seed butters, and oils) are acceptable in moderation during this plan. Although this is not a rule, I'd suggest no more than about 1-2 tablespoons of concentrated plant fats per day. And by concentrated plant fats, I mean oils and nut or seed butters. You could eat another serving of whole nuts or seeds daily, especially if you were closer to the 1 tablespoon range of concentrated plant fats.

• You may also eat whole grain flours and their products, although it's best not to overdo it if you're trying to lose weight. However, sprouted whole grain breads and tortillas can be eaten a little more liberally, as they're so high in fiber and contain very high levels of nutrients. Some examples are the "Food For Life" (Ezekiel 4:9) sprouted grain breads and sprouted grain tortillas.

• Tofu and seitan are allowed in moderation during this plan, although tempeh is preferable.

• Salty plant-based seasonings (such as tamari and miso) are healthy, as long as you don't overdo it!

• Nondairy milks (especially unsweetened) are fine in moderation during this program.

• Have a sweet tooth? No problem! A modest amount of natural sweeteners (such as agave nectar, brown rice syrup, maple syrup, or organic sugar) are acceptable in moderation—just don't eat more than one small sweet treat daily (such as pancakes with maple syrup or a small "green" or "blue" dessert).

General Do's:

• Eat only until level three of the hunger and fullness gauge (p. 12).

• Make sure you're staying up on your vegetable and water intake—it will help you fill up on fewer calories while simultaneously ensuring that you're nourished and well hydrated.

• Be kind and gentle with yourself. I probably shouldn't be telling you this, but some of my most successful clients didn't always follow this plan as well as they ideally wanted to. However, the one thing they all had in common was that they didn't give up and kept doing their best!

Two-Week Dont's

These "foods" get a big thumbs down:

• Please avoid the following: meat, poultry, fish, eggs, dairy products, and any foods that contain animal products (including gelatin, whey, fish oils, chicken broth, casein, egg whites, lamb eyes, etc.).

• Also off limits are hydrogenated (and partially hydrogenated) oils; alcoholic beverages; soft drinks; caffeine/coffee (green tea and yerba mate are acceptable substitutes); aspartame (and other artificial sweeteners); high fructose corn syrup; cornstarch (use arrowroot instead); artificial colors or flavors; preservatives; MSG; refined white sugar; and deep-fried foods.

• Whole foods (brown rice versus white rice, for example) should be emphasized over refined foods.

Two-Week Inner Wellness Basics

As you may have noticed on p. 17, I've also included some quick ways to boost your inner wellness while on this program. Because, in all honesty, being fit and healthy is great—but it won't make you truly happy unless you also have a foundation of wellness within. For those of you who are new to working on your inner selves, it really doesn't have to be all that difficult. I've tailored this program for the newbie—one who isn't used to meditating for long hours or spending half their days visualizing white light and sparkly rainbows.

Here are the inner wellness basics for the plan, as well as a little more information on each of them.

- **Look in the mirror once each day and say "I love myself" to your reflection.**

  One of the most helpful and empowering things you can do only takes about ten seconds. If you can look at yourself in the mirror every day and feel a greater and greater love for yourself, you will soon become aware of how powerful this practice is. Self-love is a natural motivator, since we automatically treat the ones we love with kindness, respect, and care. By choosing to love yourself unconditionally, you will begin to experience life with a newfound gentleness and deeply soothing peace. You will also become open to greater levels of joy and your life will automatically transform for the better.

  However, if this phrase ("I love myself") is too challenging to say to yourself at first, you can instead say "I am willing to love myself more." Even the most self-critical people (hi, I'm one) can usually do that! Looking into the mirror is such a simple—yet incredibly powerful—way to become attuned to a higher state of consciousness.

- **Think of at least five things you are grateful for each morning or evening.**

  Gratitude is one of those magical qualities that can make miracles happen. When we are in a state of gratitude, it's almost as if we become a magnet, inviting more goodness to come to us. In fact, there's something almost mysterious about the quality of gratitude. Being genuinely thankful can create miracles and dramatic shifts in energy. It is, simply put, one of the easiest ways to transform our lives. We've all heard the question: "Is your glass half full or half empty?" When we strive to see our glass as half full at all times, we somehow attract the pitcher of abundance which is waiting to fill our glass to overflowing!

- **Visualize being the ideal version of yourself.**

The practice of visualization is hands down one of the most powerful ways to change your life. Even Albert Einstein was noted for saying "Imagination is more important than knowledge." This simple quote illustrates that it's more important to have a clear vision of what you truly want than to focus on what's present in your life right now. Simply visualizing what you want will automatically align you with it and assist you in manifesting it with ease.

As a very basic example of this, I used to teach a meditation class in which everyone made a weekly commitment to themselves. One woman was really struggling with this as she kept "failing" the assignment she had given herself, which was to meditate for ten minutes each morning. Finally, after two weeks, I asked her to give up on her commitment to meditate. I suggested she instead commit to simply visualizing herself meditate. The next week, she returned to class with a very pleased look on her face. I asked her how her new assignment went. She replied that after only three days of visualizing, she had automatically (and effortlessly) started meditating for *thirty* minutes each morning! How cool is that? Additionally, visualization not only works for changing your habits—it will help you manifest a healthy, fit body as well as the life you desire. Just try it! You'll be amazed at how powerful it is when you give it a chance.

- **Meditate for at least five minutes (or sit quietly and observe your thoughts).**

Meditation is such a powerful practice! It can restore you to a state of peace and happiness and align you with your inner wisdom and intuitive self. It will help you overcome any challenging problems in your life with ease and grace and smooth out your emotions. When you're meditating on a regular basis, it's much easier to choose forgiveness over anger, love over hate, and peace over fearfulness. Simply put, meditation is the universal answer that lies within us all.

To begin meditating, I recommend starting out with a doable amount of time (such as 5-15 minutes) and building your practice from there. Also, you'll want to find a comfortable, quiet space in your home and make it as inviting as possible. There are many different methods of meditation, but I will outline three of my favorites here:

Relaxation Station

This is a good type of meditation for relieving stress and also for healing yourself if you have any ailments. Begin by allowing all of your muscles to relax completely. Start with your toes and slowly work all the way up to the top of your head (crown), allowing all of the stress to melt away in each area as you go. Although many practitioners of meditation begin with the head and work their way down, I encourage you to try it this way, as working your way *up* the body will help you maintain a higher state of consciousness.

After you have relaxed all of your muscles, think of the most beautiful color of light you can imagine. See that beautiful light filling your toes and feet completely. Next, bring that beautiful, healing light slowly upward through every part of your body until you are totally saturated in that light from toe to head. Be as open as you can, and really feel the healing energies of that light in each part of your body. Send extra light and love to any part of your being that needs it and continue to be open to healing on all levels. Enjoy this state of peace and relaxation for as long as you like. Or longer.

Affirmative Breath Meditation

This was a lifesaver for me during a really rough time in college. I had been suffering from intense anxiety attacks and was trying desperately to change my state of consciousness through meditation, affirmations, and visualization techniques. I still remember the elation I felt when I realized that this was actually working!

One way to use this method is to create a phrase based on something negative that you want to let go of, along with something positive that will replace it. Then, coordinate that phrase with your breathing. For example, I used to think "I let all darkness go" as I exhaled and "I allow light and healing" as I inhaled. Alternatively, you can use this breathing affirmation in a solely "positive" way. For example, you could think "only love flows to me" as you inhale and "only love flows from me" as you exhale. Simply choose whatever works best for you right now. You can always change it at any point if you need to. Finally, it also helps to keep your palms in an upright position as you do this exercise as it will help you maintain an increasingly receptive state of mind.

Observational Meditation

This is similar to a practice that is referred to as transcendental meditation. Begin by allowing your body to relax. Next, imagine that you are sitting inside your forehead, back toward the pineal gland. You are now an observer, viewing the activity of your mind. As if you were watching a movie, simply view your thoughts and mental images as if they were on a screen. Don't judge yourself or the images—just be *aware* of them. Get familiar with what is going on in your consciousness. Once you master this practice, it can be used at any time (and before longer meditations) to instantly produce clarity and understanding. Yes, it really is that magical!

Ready, Set, Go!

By now you're well on your way to success! You've read through this chapter and familiarized yourself with the basics of the Two-Week Wellness Solution. You've decided that you want to make some powerful, positive changes in your diet and life. Yay! However, before you begin, I'd like to recommend that you also read through the "FAQ" chapter on p. 45 as well as go through the following checklist:

√ Take a few moments to reflect before you begin. Write down a list of reasons why you're choosing to follow this program and what your goals are, *exactly*. It's also helpful to take stock of your current health before beginning. Make a note of what you weigh, how you feel, and any other current health or wellness concerns. The journal planner on p. 27 is a great place to start—plus, it will help you stay motivated if you keep it in a visible spot and look at it daily.

√ Make a list of all the recipes you want to try and foods you want to incorporate (remember, you can enjoy eating at every meal, so pick foods that sound good!).

√ Make your grocery list and go shopping for all of the necessary ingredients.

√ Review the basic daily plan (pages 15-16).

√ Although this program should be perfectly safe for any health condition, I recommend consulting a knowledgeable health-care practitioner before beginning if you have any health issues or concerns.

Keep the following tips in mind:

• As with any cleansing program, it's possible that you will experience symptoms of hunger and detoxification for the first few days. However, this is simply part of the body's natural response to letting go of toxins. The amount of symptoms you experience will depend upon your level of health and what your habits were prior to beginning this cleanse. Although most people don't experience any negative side effects, the people who do usually find that their symptoms subside within a few days. They also report feeling better than ever after the initial detoxification period as well, so don't give up!

• Because of the abundance of fiber-rich foods, it's very important to drink lots of water during this time. This plan is meant to clean you out! Needless to say, you can wave goodbye to any constipation issues. But don't worry—you can still send them a postcard.

• If at any time you're hungry on the program, begin by drinking water and eating vegetables. Next, add in "green" items. If you're still hungry, you may eat any of the following: nuts (especially walnuts and almonds), avocado, sprouted grain bread with almond butter, or a "blue" recipe.

• During these two weeks, make sure to eat (at least) the recommended amount of fruits and vegetables. This means one or two cups of fruit and six cups of vegetables each day. Remember, you are an absolute veggie monster on this plan! You simply cannot eat too many fresh, organic vegetables. They will assist you greatly in your quest for wellness, weight loss, and overall health.

Good luck—I know you can do it! And please don't forget to send me your success story.

Two-Week Journal Planner

Here's a planner that can help you track your progress and stay focused. If you like, you can photocopy it, fill it out, and post it somewhere that it can't be ignored. Be sure to give yourself lots of positive reinforcement when you fulfill your goals!

In the Beginning

- General notes on my health before beginning this program: _____
_____
- My wellness goals: _____
_____
- My starting weight: _____

My Two-Week Commitments

♥ Each day, I will meditate or sit quietly (see pages 21-23) for at least five minutes (from __:__ to __:__).

♥ I will exercise a total of _____ minutes each day, for an average of _____ minutes per week.

♥ I will be grateful for _____ things upon waking each morning (see pages 20-21 for gratitude tips—you can thank me later).

♥ I will look in the mirror and force myself to see how beautiful and lovable I am once each day. I will say _____ as I look at my fabulous reflection (see p. 20).

♥ I will use my amazing, powerful imagination to visualize myself, my daily habits, and my life as I ideally wish them to be for _____ minutes each day (see p. 21). And I'll have fun doing it!

Two-Week Wellness Rock Stars
• •

The following women were kind enough not only to commit themselves wholeheartedly to the two-week program, but also to share their results with you. Overall, each of the participants lost weight and gained health, but their individual experiences were unique and inspiring. I feel so fortunate that they were all so dedicated—plus, they really made it fun! Their success stories say it all.

Danielle Schmidt

Danielle, a stay at home mom from South Bend, Indiana, was an inspiration to many of the other participants as she completely transformed her eating habits. When she decided to try the two-week plan, she weighed 270 pounds and was looking for a complete lifestyle makeover. Over the course of three weeks (she started one week earlier than the other participants), Danielle lost a whopping 25 pounds! Specifically, she lost eleven pounds the first week, another eleven pounds the second week, and three more pounds the last week. She even started a blog (www.yepijustsaidthat.com) to journal her progress and is still following this new, healthy lifestyle with fantastic results. Simply put, I could not be more proud of her!

Here's what Danielle had to say:

Before I began Tess's program, I'd had a thought in the back of my mind for a long time that I didn't feel right. I was beginning to be aware that the things I ate made me feel "toxic." I'd always loved meat and never, ever thought I'd want to become a vegan. When the thought occurred to me to try veganism, I ignored it as long as I could! However, after reading **Radiant Health, Inner Wealth**, I finally decided to do it.

Until recently, I was a meat eater with a penchant for everything bad for me. I've been overweight for about fifteen years and just wanted to feel healthy again. I have tried countless ways to lose weight and have been a part of every weight loss plan under the sun. However, after just a short while on this plan, I knew things would finally be different. For the first time in years, I began to feel as though what I was eating was helping me feel lighter physically, emotionally, and spiritually. I could tell that in just a short while on this plan, I was finally detoxing from all the junk I'd been eating for so long. The other thing that struck me was that I could eat, and eat well! I realize now that I'd been eating the same boring seven meals over and over again for years. At this point, I only wish I'd known sooner how much I could love foods that were so good for me!

In all honesty, I'm just delighted with my results. I have never, ever felt as good as I do now. My energy is so much higher, and my mood has improved tremendously! I love that I never felt hungry on this plan and there was a lot of flexibility in what I could eat. I never felt deprived. It was easy to do and easy to understand. Plus, just a few days into the plan I noticed that my hunger became trained to this new way of eating! Plus, my IBS is steadily improving, and in just these few weeks, my blood pressure went down from 135/90 to 120/85.

And now for an update! Danielle recently reported that she has now lost a total of 45 pounds in less than three months just by sticking with her healthy new vegan diet. In essence, she's following the "G.L.E.E." principles from the "After the Plan: Radiant Health for Life!" chapter (pages 187-191). Way to go, Danielle!

Here's the update Danielle recently gave me:

Things could not be better! I feel so healthy—and despite being exposed to many colds and even strep throat, I haven't gotten sick once! I've also noticed that I heal faster—I burned myself pretty bad, and am amazed at how fast it's healing. I've also had several people comment on my skin, saying that I look radiant! My PMS symptoms used to be severe, but have now dwindled down to just feeling a little less patient. Additionally, my periods are now shorter in duration and I no longer experience painful cramps the way I used to.

For the first time in a very long time I feel I am actually listening to my body. I feel like a better person. I still have a lot of weight to lose but I feel this program is something I can really stick with long term—I can actually enjoy eating and forget about dieting, which is a huge relief. I really feel I've been granted a huge favor by the Universe in finding Tess and her program.

Millisa Barron Davis

When Millisa, a 37-year-old woman from Claremont, North Carolina, came to the two-week program, she wanted to lose weight and gain health. Millisa impressed all of us with her daily diligence in journaling her food intake—plus, her enthusiasm was contagious!

Here's what Millisa had to say about her experience:

I am so happy with the results of this plan! I love the way it was laid out and I never felt like I was starving myself. In the two weeks, I lost five pounds and gained so much energy. I am getting so much more done around the house, and no longer feel winded doing simple things like climbing stairs or going to stores.

I am so in love with this plan, in fact, that I want to continue it indefinitely and make it a full life change. I am never going back to the way I was eating—no more meat, eggs, dairy, or processed food. I feel so much better since I gave them up, and there is no need to return to them now that I know you can enjoy food so much without them!

Jennie Blechman

In southwest Colorado, Jennie is known as a vibrantly healthy herbalist who radiates wellness. However, after the holidays, Jennie confided in me that she really felt like she needed a cleanse. She showed me a detox program in a popular magazine and asked for my opinion. At first glance, I knew that program would be very hard to follow—it consisted mostly of juices and only allowed for one "solid" meal, which included animal proteins. To my delight, Jennie agreed to instead try my two-week program—and as you'll soon see, she absolutely rocked it!

Here's what she had to say after completing the two weeks:

Before starting this plan, I had been feeling like something wasn't right in my body for quite some time. I was also having a really hard time in the mornings and relying too much on coffee. But now I wake up energized every day! Just a few days into the plan, I began to have more energy than

I'd had since before my daughter was born (over six years ago), which just blows me away. I feel so much lighter and less stressed by everyday things. I was also surprised that I stopped craving coffee and bread so quickly on this plan. I don't even want my usual eggs and toast in the morning!

Although I didn't even exercise, I couldn't believe how easy it was to drop about ten pounds in just these two weeks! All of my clothes are loose and I'm feeling younger and better than ever.

What's also really exciting to me is that this is the first time in my life that I've truly stuck with any kind of program like this. I really did it! And it was so much easier than other health plans I've seen. I've even found several meals that my family loves. In fact, about a week into the plan, my husband told me that he'd lost six pounds himself just by eating dinners with me! I think his exact words were: "That crazy vegan thing you're doing made *me* lose six pounds!" I also love how much money we're saving on groceries. True, I'm buying tons of organic produce, but what a difference it makes when you stop buying expensive free range meats! I feel such immense gratitude for this plan, and will always return to it when my body needs some fine tuning.

Shonna Lovett Mackelprang

When Shonna, a full-time mom from Charleston, South Carolina, began the plan, she was hoping to improve her overall health and energy levels, as well as lose about five pounds. In the two weeks, she met her goal (despite a few dairy-based cheats!) by losing the full five pounds. Shonna was another enthusiastic participant who loved the recipes and kept us all smiling!

Here's what she said:

I love that I was able to lose all the weight I'd been wanting to lose for a while now in just the two weeks! It was so much fun trying new foods, and I loved all the recipes I tried. It was great learning a new discipline. I also loved that although Tess's plan is vegan, it is still friendly to all eaters. I've been a vegetable-loving omnivore for a long time, and this program was very easy to assimilate. I plan to continue eating more of these recipes as a delicious way to stay fit.

Tracy Riley

Tracy was unlike most of the other two-weekers in that she had already been following the recipes in *Radiant Health, Inner Wealth* for several months before starting. Just by enjoying the recipes from that book, Tracy had lost 25 pounds in the four months before she began the two-week program. Her goal was to lose a few more pounds and increase her experience of health even further. Tracy, a shelter dog volunteer from Western Arkansas, was a sheer joy to work with—her generosity of spirit and excitement about the recipes was contagious!

Here's what Tracy had to say about her experience:

Before finding Tess's book, I had been a vegetarian for twelve years, and a draggy, unhealthy one for the last couple. I had gained weight, even while running. I've finally lost weight in the last four months being a happy healthy vegan. Overall, I'm just thrilled with the results of the two weeks! I like that there are a variety of food choices and wonderful recipes from many cultures—and the color-coded system makes things so easy. I appreciated that the information made me think and use my own judgment.

On the two-week plan, I lost seven pounds! But even more exciting to me, it pushed me off my weight loss plateau straight into the middle of the healthy range on the BMI table! Now I can move a few pounds in either direction and still be in the healthy range. I have also slept more soundly, and not needed or wanted naps.

I had a "light bulb" moment about four days into this plan that made it all worth it. I now truly know what it's like to hear my body speaking its needs to me—not crazy mind cravings, but true needs. My sense of smell has returned. Something that was troubling on my leg for seventeen years is now completely gone! I feel more at peace with my eating decisions—even though I've been a vegetarian for twelve years, I still wasn't totally at peace in my soul. I now have a feeling of groundedness, strength, and all around well-being. Plus, even though I've been very active for years, the loss of 32 pounds has made my running and cycling more enjoyable, and buying clothes is a good experience again.

I plan to continue to eat using the principles of *Radiant Health, Inner Wealth* and *The Two-Week Wellness Solution* for the rest of my long, healthy life. I will judge my success by the quality and quantity of my life. I, like many others, have family members that have had untimely deaths due to disease. Their lives were filled with pain, suffering and medical visits—I plan to avoid that. I feel so grateful that I've found this way of eating, and so excited to live out the rest of my life with such increased wellness!

Sheryl (Sherrie) Thompson

Sherrie came to me through the magic of the Internet, and it was easy to see from her brilliant, genuine smile that she would have a great attitude on this plan. Indeed she did, and her results were inspirational! Sherrie lost a whopping five inches (three from her waist and two from her hips) in just the two weeks, although her weight loss was only a few pounds. This, in my experience, is because she was also doing a variety of strength-building exercises, which can increase weight through a gain in muscle (muscle weighs more than fat). In other words, if she hadn't gained so much muscle, the scales would have shown even more of a decrease in weight! Sherrie was a self-described "junk-food vegetarian" before beginning this plan, but now she's a health-food vegan who has also been transforming her family's eating habits through her own good example!

Here's what Sherrie had to say after completing the two weeks:

Before starting this plan, I was a mess—arthritis, hypertension, migraines, and chronic pain thanks to an accident five years ago. I was managing fairly well, but knew I could do better. Two weeks was all it took to really start me on the road to recovery. I no longer crave unhealthy things like coffee and artificial sweeteners either. This plan was all it took, as now I can make better choices without feeling deprived. From the first time I saw Tess's recipes, I knew that this was it! I loved that I could eat on this plan—I have a guy-sized appetite, live in a food-centric region, and have been a foodie for years. Having a variety of good food available to me that didn't take hours to prepare and appealed to my family was important. There was no real need to make a separate meal for the family and that helped me stick to plan. I'm the sole vegan in a family of four.

My sugar cravings are minimal now. That has never happened, even after six months of low carbohydrate living! My energy level is outstanding, too! I'm up between 6:15 and 6:25 every morning and go full speed ahead until

10 or 11 p.m. The afternoon crash is gone. All I do when I'm feeling slow is meditate for fifteen minutes and I'm good. I also needed to get my blood pressure and weight down without medication—this plan is helping me to do that.

Sherrie recently updated me with some more good news:

I've lost another six pounds and am feeling better than ever! I want to continue down this wonderful road as I know my health will keep improving the longer I'm following this plan. I also love that there are so many "green" desserts! I can have my cobbler and stay on track without guilt or stress. That's a huge change from anything I've previously tried.

Tami Kowal

When Tami (a 43-year-old full-time mother from Seattle) began the two-week plan, she was already vegan. However, she really wanted to experience a higher level of health, as well as lose a little weight. Additionally, she wanted to reduce bloating, increase her energy level, and avoid the auto-immune diseases that were so prevalent in her family. Luckily, she had great success! And although she got on board at the last minute, I was incredibly impressed with her immediate and continued dedication. Tami fulfilled her goals through this program and has continued to be a healthy example for her family and friends.

Here's what Tami had to say after completing the plan:

I am thrilled with the results of this plan! It was realistic, enjoyable, and insightful. I actually learned new behaviors that I absolutely will carry forward in my everyday life. Within the first two days of the plan I noticed a "lightness" in my tummy area that I loved—no more of that bloated feeling that I had grown accustomed to as normal.

What I liked best was that this plan provided an easy-to-use framework from which to eat. I was already vegan, but it's easier to be a junk-food vegan than most people think. I knew my biggest problems were refined sugars and flours, and I was eager to have some support to get away from them. The choices for each segment of the day were plentiful and delicious, and they were simple to prepare and easily accessible. This program kept me focused on getting the proper servings of fruits, vegetables, whole grains, and protein each day—yet I never measured a thing. The plan has a common sense approach and that's why I've chosen to adopt it as a lifestyle.

Over the two-week period, I lost six pounds. Plus, all my pants that used to pinch no longer did—yay! Overall, I felt a lot leaner and stronger than I had in a long time—full of energy and never deprived. After experiencing how wonderful I feel off of refined sugars and flours, I now know that I won't go back to them. It's honestly the difference between feeling sickly versus feeling healthy. I think of refined stuff now and just think, "yuck!" From now on, it's only whole grains, fruits, veggies, plant protein, and the occasional healthier sweet treat for me.

I truly believe I've done myself a great service by decreasing my risk for type 2 diabetes, which runs in my family. On this plan, I also learned to listen to my body. I now know when I'm no longer hungry and I don't continue to eat to the point of being uncomfortably full. I think eating more raw foods also forced me to slow down and be more mindful while eating. Let's face it, it's hard to "inhale" a salad while we all know it's easy to inhale a plate of pasta!

My husband and kids are also eating better, even though they didn't officially sign on. I still remember the day my daughter came bounding from her bedroom wondering "what on earth smelled so delicious" when I was cooking up the "Indian Spiced Supergrain Cereal." It gave me great joy to see her eat it right up instead of her usual sugary instant oatmeal. Even my dog started begging me for fresh carrots! So, we are all so grateful!

Before completing this plan, I already knew that eating vegan was good for me, the animals, and the planet. But now I know how to make it *amazing* for me. I am eating nutrient-dense foods and they are fueling me to the brim with life, so I'm surely not going to stop such a good thing!

Rebecca A. Weaver-Gill

Rebecca, a Chicago-based woman with a demanding schedule, was looking to boost her energy, lose some weight, and manage her bipolar symptoms. She joined the team full-force, journaling her meals and progress every day. Because of her dedication, it was no surprise that she was so successful!

Here's what Rebecca had to say about her experience:

I was very surprised at how simple and easy it was to complete this plan! I'm feeling very happy, and found that the color-coded recipes made things even easier. Plus, I loved the food! Every recipe I tried was a keeper.

Overall, I lost six and a half pounds in just the two weeks, which was actually more than I had thought possible. Another benefit that surprised me was that my skin began to look great—quite a shocker, considering the usual effects of winter in Chicago!

As I was hoping, my energy is way up. Even my mood is much improved. This has also been a great way for me to become more aware of my dietary deficiencies and understand how to improve my diet. I plan to continue following the basic structure of the two-week plan as it's easy, yummy, and healthy—what's not to like? Plus, my boyfriend even began to enjoy the meals along with me!

I should also mention that at one point, in the middle of the two weeks, everyone in my office came down with a cold. Although I still caught the cold, it was noticeable how much more quickly I bounced back than my colleagues. I am looking forward to continuing this lifestyle to see what further benefits I'll enjoy!

Bobbie Rapp

Bobbie, a growing-dome educator from southwest Colorado, came to the program hoping to jumpstart her weight loss process. However, she not only lost weight but also gained many other benefits from the plan. She was another last-minute participant who immediately jumped in with full-force dedication and impressed the heck out of me!

Bobbie says:

I am absolutely delighted with the results of this program! Before beginning the two-week plan, I could practically starve myself for six months and still never lose a pound. However, to my amazement, while on this program I lost six pounds in just two weeks—nothing short of a miracle at 53 years old! I also wish I'd measured the amount of inches I'd lost, but I didn't. However, I can tell you that my pants are much looser! What I loved most about this plan was that it actually worked, and it worked without my having to feel deprived. It was great that it involved no measuring, either (except to measure out ingredients to make recipes, of course).

I now realize that dairy and meat needs to be a minor part (if any) of my diet. I also know that I don't have to feel starved or deprived to lose weight. Instead, tuning into my "honest" hunger makes me really appreciate what I'm eating. Plus, I had no idea that I could go without coffee, and it's really been no big deal. I also became aware that I used to drink beer or wine out of thirst, not out of a real desire for them.

I've also come to realize that when I do eat meat or dairy, my digestive system complains. I've developed a taste for soy cheese and soymilk for whenever that urge strikes, and they don't feel like any sacrifice at all. I would be crazy to not continue onward with this way of eating—if it works, do it! And this really does work for me.

I'm so glad I did this and I will continue with this new lifestyle. I'm so excited to get back to a healthier, stronger, more flexible body that feels like me!

Erica Hunter

Erica, a vegan college instructor from upstate New York, simply wanted to tone up and lose a little weight. She was already quite healthy going into the program, but wanted to see how much her health could further improve. Off the bat, I was impressed with Erica's determination to stick with the program and plan out her meals despite her busy schedule. Instead of making excuses (as many others in her position would), she made things work no matter what. For once, she was set on prioritizing her own wellness, rather than putting work first.

Here's what Erica said about her experience on the program:

When I came to this program, I realized that I'd been putting my own well-being on the back burner too often. I'm fairly busy and often put work first, even above my own needs. On this plan, though, I didn't have any excuses! I had to put lunches together, pack healthy snacks, and eat a proper breakfast. I really enjoyed making the time to rethink how I'd been eating.

I found that my mood was much better than it had been before starting the program. I felt happy for longer periods than I'm used to. I just felt so good and so very happy on this plan, and had much more mental clarity as well. And although I was already thin by conventional standards, I happily lost five pounds on this program. I know I lost more inches too, as I've also been gaining muscle through my workouts. My pants that were once tight are now looser, which is great!

Following this program isn't hard if you plan out what you're going to do. For me, that meant finding the recipes that looked yummy to me, shopping well, and buying foods that I know I'll want to eat. For example, I love snap peas but don't usually buy them for some reason. However, being on this program made me realize that eating well shouldn't be a chore, so I ate snap peas to my heart's content!

Alison Ronn

When Alison (a technical writer and homeschooling mom of three boys) came to the program, her main goal was simply to learn how to eat a healthy, vegan diet. Alison was yet another dedicated participant with a positive attitude that I feel so grateful to have worked with!

Here's what Alison had to say after completing the two weeks:

I'm very happy with the results of this plan—I feel as though I really learned how to make a vegan diet doable and healthy. I really loved all of the recipes, and appreciated the amount of vegetables in the program.

Aside from losing a few pounds, the improvement in my mood was remarkable. I had a gratitude-filled day like I don't ever remember having before. I can't prove it, of course, but the way I was feeling while on this plan was awesome. Another side effect that I wasn't expecting was that my period was really light, in a very noticeable way. I plan to keep going with this healthy way of eating, as I continue to discover new recipes that will help me thrive.

Sarah Wright

Sarah, a 49-year-old mother and architect from Durango, Colorado, joined the program to lose weight and gain energy. She was thrilled to report that something had finally worked to trim down her post-pregnancy waist from the birth of her son almost four years ago.

Sarah says:

Although I was exercising regularly and eating a pretty healthy diet before beginning this program, I had not been able to lose those few extra post-pregnancy inches at my waist. However, losing weight while on the two-week plan was much easier than any previous attempts. Tess's food was very satisfying and I really looked forward to every meal, as the recipes were fantastic!

Whether you're a vegan, vegetarian, or an omnivore, many points of this program are simply good habits. I enjoy the way I feel "lighter" on this program. I also appreciate the information I learned about nutrition while on this plan. Although I was at the grocery store for fresh produce a lot, I feel I saved money since I didn't go out to eat much, drink any alcohol, or pay for packaged meals, meats, or dairy while on this program.

I lost six pounds in the two weeks—which felt like even more, since I was exercising and probably built up a little muscle weight. I also lost two inches off my waist! My face looks thinner, which others have noticed as well. Losing the post-pregnancy weight especially at my waist was a pretty big deal, because I have tried so very hard to get rid of it and hadn't been able to until following this program! I wish I'd measured my hips, as I feel I lost inches there as well. Oh well, stay tuned. I'm going to continue this program to lose a little more weight and improve my energy.

A few weeks later, Sarah gave me another update:

After an additional two weeks following the basics of the program, I lost another inch off my waist, three more pounds, and have gone down a size in pants! My energy and ability to concentrate has definitely improved as well. This program has convinced me to change many of my habits for good and my health just keeps improving!

Laura Ambler-O'Sullivan

Laura, a 39-year-old woman from Buchanan, Michigan, had her hands full when she began this program! Not only is she the executive director of the March of Dimes in Northern Indiana, but she's also a full-time wife and mother. Although she participated in the program after the rest of the group was finished, she impressed me immediately with her ability to stay on track with very little support. She is truly a two-week wellness rock star!

Here is what Laura shared with me after completing the two weeks:

I'm a "weight loss, regain, and lose again" veteran—I've tried just about anything you can imagine. You name it, I've done it. Sadly, I've never been able to make the proper lifestyle changes to lose the weight in a healthy and safe way, or to keep it off. However, I absolutely loved this plan! It was not only incredibly easy, but very effective. I've been calling it "Becoming Vegan for Dummies!"

Prior to this plan, I was absolutely awful about the things I was putting into my body for fuel. Although I was diligently working out three to five times a week, I was never seeing the results I wanted—plus, I generally felt horrible almost every time I ate—my stomach was constantly killing me! Now, I feel so light overall, and when I eat I always feel great.

It didn't take long upon starting this program before I began to really feel great—and my stomach was flat so quickly I couldn't believe it! I lost seven pounds in the two weeks and am still losing weight just by keeping up this healthy lifestyle! I love that this program not only helped me to drop the weight, but has taught me how to live a much healthier life overall that will continue well past the two weeks. Plus, this plan isn't only making me healthier, it's also affecting the eating habits of my husband, son, and even my other family members as well! I love that this has inspired those I love to become healthier. I plan to continue this healthy way of eating for the rest of my life—why wouldn't I?

I should also mention that Laura has now lost a total of twelve pounds and is maintaining her ideal weight with ease. She told me recently: "I absolutely love this way of eating! The food is great, the recipes are wonderful, my health is superb, and I feel better than ever!"

Rosine Stout

Rosine owns a successful private practice in Durango, Colorado, where she works as a registered dietician and massage therapist. She was wonderful about staying active on the blog I'd set up for the testers and was such a joy to work with.

Here's what Rosine had to say:

I lost five pounds while on the two-week program, and really enjoyed the lighter feeling I had while eating this way. Interestingly, I did go off the program after the two weeks were up, and many of my previous symptoms came back. I find that this makes me want to continue with a more vegetarian way of eating, as I had such success on this program.

I experienced all kinds of benefits from following the two-week plan. My GI tract felt like it was functioning better, I felt lighter, I had less bloating, and even my eyes were brighter and clearer. I also wasn't as tired as usual. I experienced improved bowel movements, less burping and bloating, and felt better in general about what I was eating.

I also really liked the Hunger and Fullness Gauge—it's really a great tool for anyone. I find that when you eat better, you just feel better about yourself in general.

Mary-Allison Hall

Mary-Allison, an elementary school music teacher from Columbia, South Carolina was already a healthy vegan when she began this program. However, she still wanted to lose a little weight and feel lighter in general—and you guessed it, she was a success on both counts! Yet another two-week rock star.

Here's what Mary-Allison told me about her experience:

Following this plan made me really aware of what I was eating. I'm not horribly impulsive on a regular basis, but this made me even more mindful about what I was putting into my body.

While on the program, I felt much lighter in general and lost just under five pounds (I think I would have lost even more weight if I'd exercised). I also loved that my skin got softer and clearer while following this program. I did find it was important to eat the 3 p.m. meal, as I became a little too hungry when I didn't. Live and learn, right? Overall, I'm so glad I participated in this program and will continue to use it to improve my health!

FAQ (Frequently Asked Questions)

· ·

If you're a really thorough reader and have gone through the two-week plan in this book (and maybe even scoured **Radiant Health, Inner Wealth**), you might not have any questions. Oh, and by the way, if that describes you, go ahead and put some smiley stickers and stamps that say "awesome!" all over your menu planner. However, for the rest of you, this little question and answer forum might come in handy.

Isn't fish a health food?

Due to all of the hype over Omega-3 fatty acids, fish has become a very popular "health food" in the last few years. True, these essential fats are important nutrients that every body needs. However, they're also found in many plant sources such as ground flax, walnuts, algae, and hemp seed (to name just a few).

In addition, plant-based sources of Omega-3s are also considered much safer. For example, although salmon has been considered a top source of this nutrient, even the most prominent physicians have questioned its safety levels. Dr. Mehmet Oz (or Dr. Oz as he's called on television) has come up with a great solution. He suggests that we instead turn to the source (what the salmon themselves eat) to avoid over-fishing and rising mercury levels. Salmon eat spirulena algae, which has valuable DHA Omega-3s, says Dr. Oz. "You can grow algae pretty easily, and it's a much more efficient way of getting it (than from the salmon)." [1]

Another highly respected physician who knows the area of nutrition is best-selling author, Dr. John McDougall. He states that fish is high in fat and cholesterol, highly contaminated with environmental chemicals, and therefore not a health food by any means. As with all animal products, fish contains cholesterol, excess protein, and absolutely no fiber. [2]

How will I get enough calcium if I don't eat dairy products?

I find it fascinating that the societies with the highest rates of osteoporosis are those that consume the most animal products. In societies that consume little or no dairy products, this disease (wrongly linked to inadequate calcium intake) is practically unheard of. Dr. John McDougall states, "Osteoporosis is not a disease that results from too little calcium, but rather primarily from too much animal protein." He goes on to say that animal foods "rob the body of calcium and structural materials, and thus weaken bones."[3] Simply put, the less animal protein we consume, the less calcium we need.

It should also be noted that many plant foods contain loads of calcium. Sesame, quinoa, kale, and other greens are just a few examples of foods that contain very high levels of calcium. Plus, this kind can be properly absorbed, unlike dairy products that can rob the body of calcium (because of their high levels of animal protein) while they supply it.

Finally, consider this: If you believe that we live in an intelligently designed universe, how would cow's milk originally have been intended? Perhaps to feed a baby cow? Mother's milk is as natural as it gets, and contains the ideal amount of nutrients, fat, calories, and protein for the nursing mother's growing child. Milk is absolutely the perfect food, but it is intended for the baby of that mother's species. Cow's milk is perfect for baby cows, just as human mother's milk is perfect for human babies.

How will I get enough iron if I eat a vegan diet?

Although I'm constantly asked this question, it's quite ironic since veganism is the perfect solution to iron deficiencies! In my own life, I went from being borderline anemic (as an ovo-lacto vegetarian) to having high levels of iron when I gave up dairy products almost twenty ago. This makes perfect sense because meat is high in iron while dairy products contain absolutely no iron. Therefore, it's common for people to experience a drop in iron levels when they give up meat and begin eating lots of dairy. However, when the iron-free dairy foods are dropped, it becomes very easy to get plenty of iron.

Plant-based foods are naturally iron rich—especially beans, greens, tofu, sesame seeds, and pumpkin seeds (to name a few). In fact, the only supplement I'd even consider on a healthy vegan diet is vitamin B-12, and even that is stored in the body for long periods of time. However, taking an occasional B-12 supplement is a good safety precaution for anyone, whether long-time vegan or all-time meat eater.

How will I get enough protein without eating animal foods?

I wish I had a kombucha for every time someone asked me that! However, I don't. But what I do have is the answer—which is that a lack of protein really isn't a concern as long as you're consuming enough food. In fact, the question we should instead be asking is: "How can I make sure I don't eat too much protein, since excess proteins are so detrimental to my health?" Sad, but so true. People in our culture eat waaaay too much protein! Excess proteins can seriously damage our health, resulting in calcium loss, kidney damage, and liver damage.[4]

The World Health Organization has recommended that we get five percent of our calories from protein. Five percent! Even strawberries contain eight percent protein. Of course, if you are a pregnant woman, they do recommend you increase that amount to a whopping six percent. Our highest protein needs are during infancy, since babies grow and develop at warp speed. How much protein is in mother's milk? About 5 to 6.3 percent.[5]

In truth, Americans are not in trouble because of insufficient protein intake, but rather because of an excessive protein overload. Once we reduce our protein intake (which happens naturally on a healthy plant-based diet), our bodies respond with greater health. Additionally, it should be mentioned that plant-based proteins are much more easily assimilated than those from animals, and therefore far less damaging when eaten in excess. However, if you were suffering from a disease due to excessive protein intake, the first thing to do would be to eliminate animal proteins. Next, emphasizing fruits, vegetables, and whole grains (with a moderate amount of concentrated vegetable proteins such as beans, nuts, and other legumes) would help your body restore itself to proper health.

Since coffee is natural, why isn't it allowed on the plan?

Although coffee is controversial, one thing we can all agree on is that it is powerful and potent! To quote best-selling author Rebecca Wood, "How much—if any—of this power supports your well-being depends upon your constitution, current health, and individual tolerance." [6] And although coffee is natural, it does have side effects. Its acids decrease nutrient absorption and can impair liver function. Additionally, coffee consumption has been linked to vitamin B deficiencies as well as calcium and mineral shortages. Richard Weinstein, DC, author of **The Stress Effect**, states that "too much caffeine jolts the adrenal glands and stimulates overproduction of cortisol...eventually weakening the immune system." [7]

On a personal note, I can also tell you that most of my clients were coffee drinkers before they started the two-week program. However, they invariably told me that they were able to give up coffee much more easily than they'd thought—plus, their cravings for coffee diminished quickly upon starting the program.

Thems a lot of veggies! Can you give me some ideas on how to eat them all?

Although six cups a day seems like a lot, it's actually more doable than you might think. For starters, there are lots of yummy vegetable recipes in this book, such as "Raw Catalonian Kale," "Apricot-Glazed Asparagus," and "Spicy-Sweet Ginger Cabbage." A large salad (such as "Tess's Happy Salad") can pack as much as four cups of vegetables, and some carrot or celery sticks are great for on-the-go munching.

You can also easily incorporate two cups of vegetables into many entrées—stir-fries, veggie-fried rice, "Garlic Veggie Noodle Bowl, Your Way," and Indian or Thai vegetable curries are delicious examples. You can even sauté some portabella mushrooms and onions in a little tamari, garlic, and balsamic vinegar and serve them over whole wheat penne. The trick is to have fun with it and learn to love your veggies—don't make it a chore, because it doesn't have to be one!

I'm feeling weak, cranky, and low-energy. What's going on?

Chances are, you're doing a great job eating your veggies, but perhaps you're not getting enough calories or other nutrients. Please make sure that you're also eating beans and whole grains—and don't let yourself get too hungry. Several meals are scheduled in during the day for a reason! Use them. And even if you're hungry at other times during the day, it's fine to snack, snack later, then snack some more. As long as you're filling up on the good stuff (vegetables, healthy "green" choices, and an optional "blue" food daily) and not overeating, you're completely within the bounds of this plan. And remember—you can eat your six servings of veggies, restrict your evening meal, and simultaneously consume enough (but not too many) calories. This takes a little practice, but it's so worth it! I promise.

I'm craving sweets. Help me, lady!

As the body cleanses, it often craves just the thing that it's "holding on to." I know from experience that I crave sweets when my body's still doing some cleansing, but when I'm at the point of "clean" I don't crave them at all. So, if you don't give in to your sugary desires, you will stop craving sweets once your system has fully detoxified (which won't take long if you're sticking to this program).

However, there are several "green" and "blue" dessert options that won't compromise your health. It's fine to indulge in a small serving of one of those daily. You can even do what I do (when, yes, my system isn't in the perfect place) and eat one tablespoon of organic dark chocolate chips. This is a gentle approach to cravings, as you'll still cleanse while simultaneously eating a little something sweet.

Help! I want to do the plan, but I have to feed my omnivorous family too. Whazzamitodo?

If I had a penny for every time I've heard this question, I could totally buy two packs of gum (and not just any gum—I'm talking the expensive, health-food store kind). Seriously, though, this is a very legitimate concern! A large percentage of the people who have done the two-week plan have been women with families. Omnivorous families. Junk-food-lovin' families. But the good news is that there is a solution! It just takes the will and determination to prioritize your own wellness (at least for the two weeks), and a firm commitment to yourself that you'll make it work no matter what else is going on in your life.

Additionally, what has worked well for many other women in this situation has been to choose a main dish for each meal that their families would also enjoy. For example, the "Sexy Saucy Noodles," "Black-eyed Peas with Kale," and "Hearty Vegetarian Chili" have great track records as family pleasers.

For the rest of the family, you can always throw in some familiar foods at mealtime while you stick to the program. As time goes by, you'll find your family becoming more flexible, especially as you expand your repertoire of delicious, healthy meals. Another idea is to go through the "green" and "blue" recipes with them. Make a list of all the dishes you agree on and start from there. It's a big undertaking, but it really is worth it!

I want to go to the dark, snacky place really bad. Help! What do I do?

First of all, take a minute and breathe. This happens to the best of us! Next (and before you grab that candy bar), take just a few moments to have a "time out." Ask yourself why you want to "cheat." Is it that you're feeling run down? Hungry? Bored? Without judging yourself, just inquire. Whatever your answer, it's fine. Once you've determined your reason, you can go from there. Try showing yourself some understanding, kindness, and love. Is there something you can do for yourself that won't undermine your healthy efforts? For example, could you find an alternative pleasure to indulge in, such as scheduling some you-time?

Alternatively, if you're really set on having a decadent snack, you can always see if there's something allowable on the plan that will do it for you. Perhaps a "green" or "blue" dessert or snack? Look through the recipes and find something that sounds delicious. As long as you're keeping a balance and not overeating, you're not doing anything outside of the guidelines. It takes time to let go of cravings, and in the meantime you really can find a way to feel satisfied with delicious foods that won't damage your well-being.

In fact, if you've been too strict on the two-week plan, cravings can often be a signal that it's o.k. to let up a little and invite some flavor back into your life! If you've been eating plain beans and salads with vinegar, thinking it's the best way to work your two weeks, perhaps this is a chance to rethink your long-term plan of success. Take it from me, a die-hard "foodie"—I love flavor a little too much, and that's why I came up with a cleanse that incorporated lots of delicious foods into it.

For long-term success, it's important to find foods that you love and not just force-feed yourself sprouts and lima beans all day long. Work in those Mango Spring Rolls! Dive into a raw cheezcake! Make your two weeks fun, health-supporting, and delicious. Find a way to enjoy every meal! If you do this, you'll feel so satisfied, vitalized, and trim that you'll never want to give up healthy eating. And isn't that really the point?

Do all vegetables count towards the six daily servings? How about starchy vegetables like potatoes and corn?

In general, your six servings of vegetables should come predominantly from non-starchy vegetables. However, potatoes, corn, yams, and other starchy vegetables are still "green" whole foods and can be eaten on this plan when prepared in a healthy, low-fat way.

As a daily guideline, though, you may count up to one serving of starchy vegetables toward your six servings. For example, you could eat a potato, two cups of salad, two cups of "Raw Catalonian Kale," and a cup of steamed vegetables and still punch your veggie card at the end of the day.

I exercise at night. Should I eat something afterwards?

For those of you who do evening exercise (think 5:30 p.m. spin class), you can be a little more flexible in your evening meal. Feel free to have any "green" foods afterwards, not just vegetables and beans. However, please be sure to still stay up on your water and vegetable intake, as well as heeding the usual advice to eat just until you're satisfied.

Can I substitute herbal teas for the water?

Yes, as long as the herbal teas are natural, decaffeinated, and unsweetened. In fact, this is actually a great way to get in nutrient-dense things like nettles, alfalfa, mint, blueberry leaf, hibiscus, and decaffeinated green tea. I'm a big fan of drinking nutritive herbal teas for extra vitality and for their immune-boosting properties. Bring it on!

Can I drink straight juice on the two-week plan?

Straight juice, gay juice—can't we all just get along? All right, you've paid your money so I'll stop fooling around long enough to give you an answer. Although whole fruit is preferable, some juice is fine (as long as it doesn't contain sweeteners or artificial ingredients). However, to speed up weight loss and detoxification, try to stick to whole fruits and a maximum of half to one cup of juice daily. Your total fruit intake, also, should be no more than three (or four at the most) servings daily if you're aiming for weight loss.

Why do you suggest eating only beans and vegetables after the 3 p.m. meal? Is this absolutely necessary?

For maximum weight loss, this guideline has been developed as a new twist on an old fitness trainer trick that helps you drop pounds quickly and safely. Restricting fats and starches past 3 or 4 p.m. will ensure that you're burning most of your calories off before you go to bed at night (as our metabolism slows down while we sleep).

Plus, this cutoff time will help detoxify your system, as your body will have more time to cleanse each day—resulting in glowing health and wellness for you!

However, if you're too hungry (or this doesn't work for you on certain days), you'll still be rocking (and subsequently rolling) if you stick to "green" foods at dinner time. Just make sure to eat your veggies, drink your water, and eat only until you're just satisfied.

What if I get home from work late? Can I still eat dinner?

Sorry. Go to your room without dinner and swing on some vines with the wild things. No, I'm only kidding! Yes, you may eat dinner later in the evenings, if you're hungry and get home late. This is especially fine if you stick with beans and vegetables and eat only until level three of the hunger and fullness gauge. If this is a routine, however, you may wish to consider getting in ten minutes of exercise in the evenings as this will help speed up your metabolism before bed.

If there is a scheduled meal time and I'm not hungry, should I still eat?

Nope. The really important thing is to always, always listen to your body. If you're not hungry, your body is telephoning you to say that it's busy and you should try your call again later. However, the reason why there are scheduled meals in this program is so that you don't consume your calories in one or two large sittings. It's generally better for your digestion and metabolism to eat several light, healthy mini-meals. But, if you end up skipping any of the scheduled meals, just make sure to stick with the program overall by eating your veggies at some point during the day and keeping with mainly "green" foods (and only veggies and beans after the 3 p.m. meal).

Why do you suggest eating the two cups of veggies before each p.m. meal? If I combine veggies into the meals do I still have to eat them beforehand?

Starting with fresh, crunchy vegetables is a great way to get your enzymes going, which will help you digest your food better. Plus, prioritizing your vegetables by eating them first ensures that you'll get your daily six servings. Finally, their nutrient-dense, high-fiber content will help fill you up, which means you'll feel satisfied on fewer calories (and not overdo it on the rest of your meal).

However, this is not an all-or-nothing proposal! You can certainly count any vegetables you consume during the day toward your daily requirement. As long as you're somehow working your six servings of veggies into each day, you're still on the plan, kicking butt, and, yes, taking names.

Why do you suggest eating fruit in the morning? Is it o.k. to eat it later in the day?

Starting your day with lemon water and fruit is the ideal way to say "good morning" to your digestive system after your evening fast. Fruit is a nourishing, light way to really start the day off right. However, you may certainly still consume fruit later in the day if you like. Just try to stick to vegetables and beans after your 3 p.m. meal for maximum weight loss.

I've heard that a cleanse is best accomplished in the spring or fall. Is it smart to do this program in the winter?

Here's a personal experience in response to this question: The best cleansing my body ever did happened to be during the winter. However, I too had some reservations beforehand. Didn't I need the extra fat to keep me warm? Well, I realized (and this was about ten years ago) that I had been making excuses for a long time to hold onto toxins in my system. I was finally ready to make some big changes, and it just so happened to coincide with the dead of winter. So, I bought some long underwear and went for it!

However, I should mention—and this is a biggie—that this cleanse, the Two-Week Wellness Solution, is different than most others. I do not call for rigorous fasting or calorie deprivation. You can eat, eat later, and then eat some more. And yes, it's easier to find awesome, shimmery-shiny vegetables in the middle of a summertime farmer's market. But, where there's a will, there's a way! You can still find lots of healthy, happy veggies and fruits in the organic produce section of almost any health food store or supermarket.

What in blue blazes is this kombucha of which you speak?

Kombucha (or "K" as I've affectionately nicknamed it) is a fermented Chinese tea. Fizzy and very rejuvenating, it's highly detoxifying as well. Many people make their own, but there's a great brand on the market called GT Synergy. Personally, I favorite the grape, strawberry, passionberry, gingerberry, and guava flavors. One bottle of kombucha daily is fine on this program, and would be considered "green."

Why do you recommend sprouted breads and tortillas?

Anytime you sprout something (whether a grain, seed, or legume) you exponentially increase the nutrients that are available to you through that food. Think of sprouted foods as nutrition explosions, gleefully nurturing every cell of your body.

The other great thing about sprouted foods is that you're getting more whole foods (versus flours) into your system. Many sprouted grain products are even completely flour-free, which means that you're getting insanely nourished by eating only sprouted whole foods.

As far as personal recommendations, my favorite in the bread department is the "Food for Life" Ezekiel 4:9 sesame. For tortillas, I often buy the "Alvarado Street" brand, as they're still soft and pliable (as you'd like tortillas to be) but made from a combination of whole grains and sprouts. The 100% sprouted tortillas are uber-healthy, but almost impossible to bend without breaking— therefore, I use them for quesadillas or in other ways that they don't need to be, well, bent. For burritos and wraps, the Alvarado Street tortillas are ideal.

What do you consider to be one serving of vegetables or fruits?

I use the old standard, which is that one serving equals approximately one cup. Also, whole fruits are one serving, unless they're very large. For example, a whole grapefruit is two servings, while a medium orange is one serving. I consider a large carrot or large celery stalk to be one serving of vegetables as well.

As a guideline, just make sure you're getting a good variety of veggies daily that roughly add up to at least six cups. Your body will love you for it!

I have some veggie juice questions! First of all, should I use a Vitamix or regular juicer? Why do you suggest juicing the lemon peels? And can I change up the vegetables?

Either juicing device is fine. A Vitamix is great as you'll retain the fiber along with the nutrients. However, if you prefer a smoother, easier-to-drink concoction, simply use a regular juicer.

The peel of an organic lemon will add loads of nutrients and a nice, tart flavor element. However, if you can't find organic lemons, you shouldn't use the peels. Instead, simply place the juice of a regular lemon into your veggie juice once it's done.

As far as varying the veggies you juice, it's fine! Have fun and go wild. Just don't leave out the lemon (if the vegetable juice is a substitute for the a.m. lemon water).

What's the deal with stevia?

Stevia's awesome! It's a sweetener that's actually made from a healthy, whole food—green stevia leaves from the stevia plant. Fancy that! It's very concentrated, though, so a little goes a very long way.

The only drawbacks are that some don't like its bitter taste, which to me depends on how it's used. Personally, I like it in a healthy shake (or my homemade nondairy milk), for example, but not in most desserts. Also, it's best not to give young children excessive amounts of stevia, as it's been linked to inhibiting growth when consumed in large amounts. However, a moderate use of stevia in children's diets should be perfectly safe.

I'm a little confused about what makes something "green." You say not to overdo it on flour or juice, but some recipes that include them are labeled "green." What gives, sister?

Think of this program as one of those movies where the director actually trusted her audience enough to make the jokes subtle. She had enough confidence in the innate intelligence of her viewers to know that they'd figure things out. Likewise, I have no interest in designing a program that is so rigid that no one can actually follow it—or if they do, makes them want to go to the dark place on day fifteen! No. Instead, it was my goal to create a plan that had a balance of structure and freedom. That while cleansing and detoxifying the participants, would also leave them feeling satisfied and wanting to stick with their deliciously rewarding new lifestyle!

Also, not all recipes labeled "green" (or "blue," for that matter) are created equal. While sprouts and smoothies are both "green," for example, sprouts are a completely raw whole food while smoothies contain some refined juice. However, it's all about the balance! If you are eating all whole foods otherwise, your system will have no problem with some unsweetened fruit juice in your morning smoothie. Only you know what will keep you on track. Choose mostly whole foods and go light on the juice and flour-based products. And remember: This is about your life. You're laying the foundation for a healthy new way of being that you'll want to stick with long-term. Make sure it fits and that you enjoy it!

How important is it to use fresh lemon juice in my water each morning?

It's actually pretty important. The juice of fresh lemons will do wonders to detoxify, alkalinize, and cleanse your system. Bottled lemon juices are very denatured, and therefore don't do a whole lot for you. Even if you can only find non-organic fresh lemons, I still recommend using them as they're not on the list of foods to avoid if non-organic (please see p. 62). There is just nothing—**nothing**—like fresh lemon juice in the morning to get your body happily on track!

Why don't you recommend grapeseed or canola oil?

Unless you can find organic grapeseed oil, I do not recommend it. Grapes, if commercially grown, contain one of the highest levels of pesticides, which are even more concentrated in their seeds. Therefore, the oil extracted from the seeds makes for a chemical cocktail! Canola is another oil, like non-organic grapeseed, that has been marketed as a "health food" but really isn't as it's highly refined. Additionally, canola oil is considered toxic according to Chinese medicine.

What kind of milk do you recommend?

Personally, I'm gonzo over my soymilk maker. It paid for itself in about four months and now I can make unprocessed, unsweetened milk for pennies! It also makes me immensely happy to store my homemade milk in reusable glass containers. Yes, I'm easy to please!

Personally, I make a mixture that is about 40% organic soybeans, 40% almonds, and 20% brown rice (or barley or oats). I like this because it cuts down on any "over-soying" and brings in a variety of nutrients. To make the milk, I just soak all of the ingredients overnight and then pop them in the machine. It's extremely easy. There is no pre-cooking of the beans or grains, and the milk is done in fifteen minutes. I usually don't sweeten it, but sometimes do add a few drops of liquid stevia if my daughter is hankering for "sweet milk."

However, if you don't have a soymilk maker (and don't intend to buy one), there are lots of great nondairy milks on the market. Just look for a brand that contains organic ingredients and no added sweeteners. Additional recommendations are on p. 181 in the "'Green' Packaged Foods" section of this book.

Why do you call for coconut oil? Isn't that a saturated fat?

Yes, it is. But ironically, coconut oil is one of the healthiest oils you could choose. For one thing, it has very high levels of medium-chain fatty acids, the kind that are not stored as fat in the body. Furthermore, coconut oil has been shown to improve metabolism and immune system function.

The reason coconut oil got its reputation as a bad guy was because it had always been studied along with animal fats as part of a saturated fat group. Once coconut oil parted ways with the offending party (lard) and was studied on its own, it was found to be innocent of all charges.

Do I have to give up my coffee, glass of wine, and all animal foods for this to work?

I know it's hard, but yes. Tell yourself that it's just two weeks. You can do anything for two weeks, right? After the program, you can reevaluate your needs and desires and go from there. And for those of you who have a coffee addiction, try yerba mate, green tea, or kombucha. They still have some caffeine, but are much milder and are also rich in health-supporting antioxidants.

Why do you call for both extra-virgin and regular for the olive and coconut oils?

Although the extra-virgin variety of both is the healthiest choice, you don't always want your food to taste like olives or coconut. For those times when you just need a neutral-flavored oil, the non-virgin varieties of both are your healthiest choices.

What if I need more sustenance first thing in the morning than just the lemon water and fruit?

As always, this plan can be made to fit with your lifestyle. Only you know what will really make this a healthy, thriving discipline in your life. So, if necessary, you can instead eat your one or two servings of fruit later in the day. After your lemon water, you may have any of the following:

• Whole grain hot cereal with nondairy milk (or a raw, sprouted cereal)

• A high-fiber, vegan breakfast cereal (preferably organic and containing at least six grams of fiber per serving)

• A piece of sprouted grain toast with almond butter and jam or agave nectar (this would be a "blue" option)

• A power shake (such as the "Super Shake-A-Go-Go") or smoothie work great! They'll give you loads of sustenance, while still allowing you to get in your fruit requirement first thing.

I'm on a budget—do I need expensive gadgets, a juicer, special foods, or other expensive whatnots to do this?

That's up to you. If you want to full-on chef it up, you can run to the store and buy everything from hemp protein powder to a soymilk maker to a dual-sided blender. However, **you** choose what recipes you want to incorporate into your menu. You can be 110% successful on this plan just by eating simply and making smarter choices at your regular grocery store.

What if I get really hungry?

Eat. You can have unlimited "green" foods and one "blue" food daily. However, the rule of thumb if you're hungry outside of mealtime is to start by drinking some water. Next, make sure you're up on your veggie intake (you're going for at least six cups daily). Finally, if you're still hungry, listen to your body. It will tell you what it needs.

I'm going to be very busy. Can I still do the plan?

Yes! You can make this program totally on-the-go friendly. Only a little planning and forethought are necessary. I recommend carving out a little time before you begin to write out your weekly plan and menu. Be sure to emphasize quick, easy recipes and keep your schedule in mind. To ensure that you'll be eating well when you don't have time to cook, you can also check out the "'Green' Packaged Foods" (on pages 181-185) for healthy packaged items. And remember—where there's a will there's always a way!

What if I get really hungry when I'm on the go?

Many healthy choices can be made. For example, a rice cake, some nuts, or a piece of fruit often do the trick quite nicely, and they are available in any grocery store. In general, snacking is not a problem unless you're making poor choices or eating past the point of feeling just satisfied (level three on the hunger and fullness gauge, p. 12). Also, you can use this as an opportunity to plan better so that in the future you're well prepared with healthy snacks when you're out and about.

What if I have to go to one of those restaurant-type places during the two weeks?

Whether you've been dragged to a Mexican restaurant or your favorite steak house, you can usually still find some (relatively) healthy choices. Some examples are a bean tostada, steamed vegetables, or a large salad with kidney or garbanzo beans. Are there any healthy, whole food choices on the menu, such as a baked potato, vegan soup, or veggie stir-fry? Buddy up to your server and ask questions. Do they use lard, eggs, or other animal-based ingredients? Would the chef be willing to make you a special item?

And if going to a restaurant makes you want to eat crazy, remind yourself that it's just for two weeks—you can come back when the plan's over and pig out. Although, chances are that you'll be feeling so good after completing the program that you won't want to!

Does all my food have to be organic now?

Before you freak out about the million dollar grocery bills that organic produce will rack up, I urge you to relax. Have a cup of tea. Breathe and smile. Sit down and put your feet up. . . while you check this crazy madness out:

Researchers at Rutgers University conducted a study a few years ago where they purchased both non-organic and organic versions of the same fruits and vegetables at a supermarket. They then analyzed them to see how their nutritional profiles compared. The findings were absolutely amazing! Not only were the organic foods higher in nutrients, but they were so by huge percentages!

Here are just a few examples of their findings: [8]

- Lettuce take this for example: Inorganic lettuce contained 9 trace elements parts per million dry matter (tep) of iron while the organic version contained a whopping 516 tep!

- Tomatoes: While the inorganic tomatoes registered at 1 tep for iron, the organic tomatoes came in at 1938.0 tep of iron! Sheer madness.

• Spinach: Our fine friend potassium is present in non-organic spinach in the amount of 84.6 millequivalents per 100 grams dry weight (mpg). In organic spinach, potassium registers at 237.0 mpg. Known for its high iron content, spinach (when grown conventionally) registers at 19 tep for iron. However, organic spinach came in at 1,584 tep! No, that's not a misprint.

All things considered, to get the most out of your foods, it's clear that organic is the best choice. Still, if switching to an exclusively organic diet overnight sounds intimidating, you can begin by first phasing out the foods that are the most contaminated.

So, here's a supermarket cheat-sheet you can use—which will also come in handy when everything isn't available organically and you need to make some informed choices.

Supermarket Organics Cheat-Sheet:

Foods that should only be eaten if organic (most contaminated when non-organic): [9]

Apples, bell peppers, celery, cherries, grapes, nectarines, peaches, pears, potatoes, spinach, strawberries, green beans, tomatoes, lettuces, citrus zest, Mexican cantaloupe, and apricots. Notice a trend here that includes many thin-skinned fruits and veggies.

Foods that are the least contaminated when non-organic: [10]

Asparagus, avocados, broccoli, sweet corn, kiwi, mango, onions, papayas, pineapples, sweet peas, blueberries, Brussels sprouts, cabbage, eggplant, oranges, grapefruits, okra, plums, radishes, bananas, and watermelon. Notice that several of these "safer" non-organic items are tropical fruits.

A Comprehensive Two-Week Plan

• •

Not so keen on the planning? Then this chapter should make you smile. It includes everything you'll need to rock the two-week plan—a complete menu, shopping list, and even do-ahead food preparation tips. However, keep in mind that this is only meant as a helpful option for you—you are totally free to make up your own menu, as long as you stick with the basic guidelines of the plan.

I've also found that it's nice to have a sample plan to look at, as it shows you just how much flavor and food you can enjoy while still cleansing and losing weight. By no means should your journey to ultimate wellness be bland and boring! Plus, you'll stick with the plan more easily (and want to keep it going after the two weeks) if you incorporate lots of foods that you truly enjoy.

When using this plan, please keep in mind that it's set up for just one person. However, you can multiply the ingredients to feed more people if need be. For ideas on feeding a not-so-compliant family while you're cruising on the two-week plan, please see pages 49-50.

WEEK ONE

Day 1

Breakfast:
Lemon water (p. 84)
"Sunshine Smoothie" (p. 91)

Mid-morning:
Small bowl of high-fiber cereal (p. 182) with nondairy milk

Lunch:
Two cups baby greens with "Light Balsamic Dressing" (p. 128)
One slice "Springtime Bruschetta" (p. 107)
One cup "Low-Fat Basil Garlic Linguine" (p. 166)

3 p.m. mini-meal:
One cup steamed cauliflower
"Spicy Sweet Potato Fries" (p. 131)

Dinner:
Carrots and celery sticks (two cups worth)
"Black-eyed Peas with Kale" (p. 162)

Day 2

Breakfast:
Lemon water (p. 84)
Piece of fresh fruit

Mid-morning:
"Cranberry-Lime Confetti Quinoa" (p. 106)

Lunch:
"Spinach Strawberry Salad" (p. 117)
One "Triathlon Tostada" (p. 154)
"Zingy Grilled Orange-Ginger Grapefruit" (p. 172)

3 p.m. mini-meal:
"Oven Roasted Cauliflower with Rosemary and Garlic" (p. 99)
(half of the batch)
One "Shiitake-Basil Spring Roll" with "Thai Skinny Dipping Sauce" (p. 136)

Dinner:
Carrots and celery (two cups worth)
"Ful Mudhamas" (p. 157)

Day 3

Breakfast:
Lemon water (p. 84)
½ grapefruit

Mid-morning:
"Ful Mudhamas" (p. 157)

Lunch:
Two cups baby greens with "Light Balsamic Dressing" (p. 128)
One slice "Springtime Bruschetta" (p. 107)
One cup "Low-Fat Basil Garlic Linguine" (p. 166)

3 p.m. mini-meal:
"Oven Roasted Cauliflower with Rosemary and Garlic" (p. 99), the rest from day 2
One "Shiitake-Basil Spring Roll" with "Thai Skinny Dipping Sauce" (p. 136)

Dinner:
One cup celery sticks
"Black-eyed Peas with Kale" (p. 162)

Day 4

Breakfast:
"Veggie Vitality Juice," using parsley as your greens (p. 85)

Mid-morning:
Fruit salad (1 cup of berries with one sliced banana)

Lunch:
Two cups baby greens with "Light Ginger-Miso Dressing" (p. 128)
Two "Triathlon Tostadas" (p. 154)

3 p.m. mini-meal:
"Spicy Sweet Potato Fries" (p. 131)
One "Shiitake-Basil Spring Roll" with "Thai Skinny Dipping Sauce" (p. 136)

Dinner:
Two cups steamed cauliflower
"Black-eyed Peas with Kale" (p. 162)

Day 5

Breakfast:
Lemon water (p. 84)
½ grapefruit

Mid-morning:
"Spinach Strawberry Salad" (p. 117)

Lunch:
One carrot, cut into sticks
One slice "Springtime Bruschetta" (p. 107)
One cup "Low-Fat Basil Garlic Linguine" (p. 166)

3 p.m. mini-meal:
Two "Shiitake-Basil Spring Rolls" with "Thai Skinny Dipping Sauce" (p. 136)
½ cup "Zen Rice with Seaweed Gomasio" (p. 103)

Dinner:
Two cups steamed cauliflower
"Get Skinny Soup" (p. 146)

Day 6

Breakfast:
"Veggie Vitality Juice," using parsley as your greens (p. 85)

Mid-morning:
"Sunshine Smoothie" (p. 91)

Lunch:
Two cups baby greens with "Light Balsamic Dressing" (p. 128)
"Ful Mudhamas" (p. 157)
"Cranberry-Lime Confetti Quinoa" (p. 106)
"Zingy Grilled Orange-Ginger Grapefruit" (p. 172)

3 p.m. mini-meal:
"Spinach Strawberry Salad" (p. 117)
One "Triathlon Tostada" (p. 154)

Dinner:
One cup raw veggies (carrots or celery)
"Black-eyed Peas with Kale" (p. 162)

Day 7

Breakfast:
Lemon water (p. 84)
Piece of fresh fruit, your choice

Mid-morning:
"Ful Mudhamas" (p. 157)

Lunch:
"Spinach Strawberry Salad" (p. 117)
One slice "Springtime Bruschetta" (p. 107)
One cup "Low-Fat Basil Garlic Linguine" (p. 166)

3 p.m. mini-meal:
One cup baby greens with "Light Ginger-Miso Dressing" (p. 128)
"Spicy Sweet Potato Fries" (p. 131)
One "Triathlon Tostada" (p. 154)

Dinner:
Carrots and celery sticks (two cups worth)
"Get Skinny Soup" (p. 146)

Note: If you don't have a juicer. . .

Simply substitute lemon water and a piece of fruit for the vegetable juice on the days that call for a morning veggie juice. On those days, you'll also need to fit in an extra serving of vegetables at some point. Finally, you'll need to adjust your shopping list accordingly by buying a few extra servings of fruit and not purchasing the items needed for the juice (those modifications are noted on the shopping list for your convenience).

Shopping List Week One:

This is everything you'll need for week one. It may look like a lot, but keep in mind that this list was made as if you were starting from ground zero! In other words, this list would be the same if you were living on the beach, without even a spare mango in your tent. Many of you may already have most of these items on hand—and if you don't, they make great additions to your pantry. But don't worry, next week you'll have less to buy—and less to prepare—as much of what you buy (and do) will carry over. Happy shopping!

PRODUCE YOU'LL NEED:

- Two grapefruits
- Fifteen lemons
- Two organic lemons (only purchase if you have a juicer—these should be organic, as their skins will be used)
- Six limes
- Large bunch parsley
- One bunch kale (lacinato if available)
- Three bananas
- One pint strawberries
- 5 oz. bag baby spinach
- Two mangoes
- Two pieces of fresh fruit (your choice—go crazy)
- Four large heads (bulbs) of garlic (41 cloves worth)
- One organic orange
- 2 lb. bag of carrots
- One bunch of celery
- Four tomatoes (purchase only two if you don't have a juicer)
- Twelve cups of baby greens
- Green cabbage (one head)
- Two onions (white or yellow)
- Fresh ginger root
- Two avocados
- Three small sweet potatoes
- Fresh basil (the equivalent of two cups, packed)
- One bunch of cilantro
- One package/bunch of green onions (scallions)
- One head of cauliflower

- Fresh rosemary
- Three cups of shiitake mushrooms (you may instead purchase these in the frozen section if you can find them there—a good brand is "Woodstock Farms")

FROZEN FOODS/MISCELLANEOUS ITEMS YOU'LL NEED:

- Bag of frozen berries (or a carton of fresh berries)
- One package of sprouted grain (or whole grain) bread (made without refined flours—the Ezekiel breads are a good choice)
- One package of organic corn tortillas (preferably made with sprouted corn)

STAPLES/PANTRY ITEMS YOU'LL NEED:

- High-fiber whole grain dry cereal (at least six grams of fiber per serving—please see "'Green' Packaged Foods" on pages 181-185 for ideas)
- 8 oz. package of whole grain pasta (preferably linguine, but any shape works)
- One package of bean thread noodles (or thin rice noodles), available in the Asian food section of most supermarkets and health food stores
- One package of spring roll wraps (these are very fragile, white in color, and made mainly from rice and/or tapioca—they're available in the Asian food section of most supermarkets and health food stores)
- One package of dry quinoa (whole quinoa grain), the regular tan-colored variety
- One package of dry red quinoa (whole quinoa grain)
- One package of long grain brown rice
- One 15 oz. (or 14.5 oz.) can of crushed tomatoes
- One 14.5 oz. can of diced tomatoes with garlic and onions
- One 14.5 oz. can of low-fat coconut milk
- Natural peanut butter
- Agave nectar
- One cup dry lentils (plain old brown lentils, like your mama used to cook with—or at least my mama)
- One and a half cups dry black-eyed peas
- Crystallized ginger
- Nondairy milk (unsweetened and organic)
- Orange juice (not from concentrate)
- Two 15 oz. cans of pinto beans (or fava beans)

- One 15 oz. can of black beans
- All-purpose oil (sunflower, non-virgin olive, or non-virgin coconut)
- Extra-virgin olive oil
- Coconut oil
- Mellow white miso
- Toasted (dark) sesame oil
- Organic sugar
- Optional: Sriracha Sauce (the kind with a rooster on the front of the bottle—if you like, you can substitute cayenne powder or simply omit)
- Tamari (or shoyu or organic soy sauce)
- Balsamic vinegar
- Apple cider vinegar
- Pure maple syrup
- Poppy seeds
- Two cups of sesame seeds (regular)
- Optional: small package of black sesame seeds
- One cup sliced (or slivered) almonds
- Bottled hot sauce of your choice (such as tabasco)
- Dried cranberries, unsulphured

SPICES/SEASONINGS YOU'LL NEED:

- Sea salt
- Black pepper
- Turmeric
- Cayenne powder
- Cumin powder
- Oregano
- Onion granules (granulated onion; a grainier version of onion powder)
- Bay leaves
- Kombu (available in any self-respecting health food store, see p. 147)
- Nori (available in square sheets in health food stores)
- Nutritional yeast powder (found in health food stores)
- Seasoned salt
- Garlic granules (kind of like garlic powder, but grainier—think "tiny edible garlic sand particles")
- Celery seed
- White pepper
- Lemon-pepper

- Dried dill
- Dried rosemary
- Paprika
- Dulse flakes (available in health food stores)
- Kelp powder (available in health food stores)

Prepare for Greatness!

Do-Ahead Tips for Week One:

Setting aside the time to do some food preparation in advance makes for much less work at mealtime. For many, a designated day (such as Sunday) works well for this purpose. If you do take the time to prepare these items in advance, you'll find it makes your life much easier when everyone's hungry!

Here's another tip: If possible, get your bananas in advance—that way the ones you'll be freezing for smoothies will have a chance to ripen. However, if you can buy them when they're already very ripe, you can freeze them right away. This, incidentally, is one of my favorite grocery "scores." If you play your cards right, you can sometimes find extra-ripe bananas marked way down. To me, it's the perfect equation! Ripe, ready-to-freeze bananas + a fat discount = happiness.

Make in advance:

1. "Light Balsamic Dressing" (p. 128)
2. "Thai Skinny Dipping Sauce" (p. 136)
3. "Light Ginger-Miso Dressing" (p. 128)
4. "Seaweed Gomasio" (p. 124)

Optional make-ahead items:

1. "Cranberry-Lime Confetti Quinoa" (p. 106)
2. "Get Skinny Soup" (p. 146)
3. You can prepare the individual items for the "Shiitake-Basil Spring Rolls" (p. 136) and store them separately in airtight containers in the fridge.
4. Pre-bake your tostada shells (once cooled, store in an airtight container) and prepare the bean mixture for "Triathlon Tostadas" (p. 154).
5. Cut your cauliflower into florets and refrigerate in an airtight container.
6. Prepare your carrots and celery. . . for their demise.

WEEK TWO

Day 8

Breakfast:
Lemon water (p. 84)
Piece of fresh fruit, your choice

Mid-morning:
Small slice "Lemon Coconut Vanilla Bean Cheezcake" (p. 170)

Lunch:
One "Vietnamese Spring Roll" (p. 140)
"Sexy Saucy Noodles" (p. 159)

3 p.m. mini-meal:
Two cups baby greens with "Light Balsamic Dressing" (p. 128)
One "Triathlon Tostada" (p. 154)

Dinner:
"Cucumber Dill Toss" (p. 114)
"Lickety Split Pea Soup" (p. 147)

Day 9

Breakfast:
Lemon water (p. 84)
Fruit salad (raspberries and a banana)

Mid-morning:
Small bowl of high-fiber cereal (p. 182) with nondairy milk

Lunch:
Two cups baby greens with "Light Ginger-Miso Dressing" (p. 128)
"Baked Chimichanga" (p. 156) with "Kid's Choice Guacamole" (p. 100)

3 p.m. mini-meal:
Two "Vietnamese Spring Rolls" (p. 140)
½ cup "Zen Rice with Seaweed Gomasio" (p. 103)

Dinner:
Two cups raw veggies, your choice
"Get Skinny Soup" (p. 146)
"Five-Minute Five-Bean Salad" (p. 115)

Day 10

Breakfast:
Lemon water (p. 84)
Piece of fresh fruit, your choice

Mid-morning:
Small slice "Lemon Coconut Vanilla Bean Cheezcake" (p. 170)

Lunch:
Two cups baby greens with "Light Ginger Miso Dressing" (p. 128)
"Lickety Split Pea Soup" (p. 147)
Optional: one serving "Zen Rice with Seaweed Gomasio" (p. 103)

3 p.m. mini-meal:
One "Vietnamese Spring Roll" (p. 140)
"Sexy Saucy Noodles" (p. 159)

Dinner:
"Cucumber Dill Toss" (p. 114)
"Five-Minute Five-Bean Salad" (p. 115)

Day 11

Breakfast:
"Veggie Vitality Juice," using parsley as your greens (p. 85)

Mid-morning:
"Sunshine Smoothie" (p. 91)

Lunch:
Two cups baby greens with "Light Balsamic Dressing" (p. 128)
"Baked Chimichanga" (p. 156) with "Kid's Choice Guacamole" (p. 100)

3 p.m. mini-meal:
"Garlic Veggie Noodle Bowl, Your Way" (p. 158, with rice noodles and broccoli)

Dinner:
2 cups steamed Brussels sprouts with "Fat-Free Maple Dijon Dressing" (p. 126)
"Get Skinny Soup" (p. 146)

Day 12

Breakfast:
Lemon water (p. 84)
Mango raspberry fruit salad (1 mango and 1 cup raspberries)

Mid-morning:
Small bowl of high-fiber cereal (p. 182) with nondairy milk

Lunch:
One "Vietnamese Spring Roll" (p. 140)
"Sexy Saucy Noodles" (p. 159)

3 p.m. mini-meal:
One medium carrot, cut into sticks
One "Vietnamese Spring Roll" (p. 140)
"Lickety Split Pea Soup" (p. 147)
One slice "Quick and Healthy Herbed Garlic Bread" (p. 104)

Dinner:
"Cucumber Dill Toss" (p. 114)
"Five-Minute Five-Bean Salad" (p. 115)

Day 13

Breakfast:
"Veggie Vitality Juice," with parsley (p. 85)

Mid-morning:
"Berry Good Morning Shake" (p. 90, made with raspberries)
Optional: Small bowl of high-fiber cereal (p. 182) with nondairy milk

Lunch:
Two "Vietnamese Spring Rolls" (p. 140)
"Garlic Veggie Noodle Bowl, Your Way" (p. 158, with rice noodles and broccoli)

3 p.m. mini-meal:
"Baked Chimichanga" (p. 156) with "Kid's Choice Guacamole" (p. 100)

Dinner:
Two cups raw veggies, your choice
"Get Skinny Soup" (p. 146)

Day 14

Breakfast:
Lemon water (p. 84)
One piece of fresh fruit, your choice
Optional: Small bowl of high-fiber cereal (p. 182) with nondairy milk

Mid-morning:
Small slice "Lemon Coconut Vanilla Bean Cheezcake" (p. 170)

Lunch:
Two cups Brussels sprouts with "Fat-Free Maple Dijon Dressing"
(p. 126)
"Five-Minute Five-Bean Salad" (p. 115)
One slice "Quick and Healthy Herbed Garlic Bread" (p. 104)

3 p.m. mini-meal:
Two "Vietnamese Spring Rolls" (p. 140)
"Sexy Saucy Noodles" (p. 159)

Dinner:
"Cucumber Dill Toss" (p. 114)
"Lickety Split Pea Soup" (p. 147)

Shopping List Week Two:

PRODUCE YOU'LL NEED:

- Nine lemons
- Three pieces of fresh fruit, your choice
- Three bananas
- Two mangos
- Two large organic lemons
- Two limes
- Eight cups of baby greens
- Four cups of Brussels sprouts
- One large bunch of broccoli
- Two cups of shiitake mushrooms (you may instead purchase these frozen)
- Four cups of raw veggies, your choice
- Two tomatoes
- One package of bean sprouts
- One bunch of fresh parsley
- Two lbs. of carrots
- Two medium-large cucumbers
- One medium red onion
- Fresh dill (¼ cup worth)
- One bunch of celery
- Three heads (bulbs) of fresh garlic (25 cloves)
- Fresh ginger root
- One bunch of cilantro
- Romaine lettuce
- One package/bunch of scallions (green onions)
- One avocado

FROZEN FOODS/MISCELLANEOUS ITEMS YOU'LL NEED:

- One package of frozen edamame (shelled)
- Two packages of frozen raspberries
- One package of firm, water packed tofu (refrigerated)
- One package of whole grain (or sprouted) tortillas
- Your favorite salsa (preferably the fresh, refrigerated variety)

STAPLES/PANTRY ITEMS YOU'LL NEED:

- One package of buckwheat soba noodles (usually about 12 oz. in size)
- Hoisin Sauce (available in the Asian food section of most supermarkets and health food stores)
- One package of rice noodles (or corn-quinoa spaghetti) for the "Garlic Veggie Noodle Bowl, Your Way"
- One bottle of Thai spicy chili sauce (I use "Thai Kitchen" brand)
- One cup of green split peas (dry)
- One cup of pinto beans (dry)
- One 15 oz. can of garbanzo beans
- One 15 oz. can of mixed beans (or other beans of choice such as kidney or pinto)
- One cup whole almonds (untoasted)
- Small bag of dates
- Raisins
- Cashews
- Coconut butter (not oil)
- One vanilla bean
- Vanilla extract
- Dijon mustard

SPICES/SEASONINGS YOU'LL NEED:

- Yellow mustard powder
- Dried basil

Prepare for Greatness!

Do-Ahead Tips for Week Two:

Please see the banana tips on p. 71 and keep them in mind for this week.

Make in advance:

1. Make the "Lemon Coconut Vanilla Bean Cheezcake" (p. 170). To keep yourself on the straight and narrow, cut it into twelve slices and then freeze each piece individually. From there, you can remove one slice at a time and thaw for 30 minutes before serving.
2. "Cucumber Dill Toss" (p. 114)
3. "Fat-Free Maple Dijon Dressing" (p. 126)

Optional make-ahead items:

1. You can prepare the Hoisin Sauce and the other individual items for the "Vietnamese Spring Rolls" (p. 140). They can be stored separately in airtight containers in the fridge.
2. Cut the broccoli into florets and store in an airtight container in the fridge.
3. "Lickety Split Pea Soup" (p. 147)
4. "Five-Minute Five-Bean Salad" on p. 115 (Although this is obviously very quick to make, it's even better if allowed to marinate in advance.)
5. Prepare your veggies of choice (and individually bag them if it makes you deeply happy).

Two-Week Menu and Shopping Planner

Here's a food planning guide that can be photocopied—or simply used as a tool to create your own masterful plan. Food nerds, unite!

My meal planning day: _____ **My cooking day(s):** _____

Foods for Breakfast and Mid-Morning:
- Lemon water
-
-
-

Foods for Lunch and the 3 p.m. Meal:
-
-
-
-
-

-
-
-
-
-

Foods for Dinner and After 3 p.m. (Beans and Veggies):
-
-
-
-

-
-
-
-

Shopping Guide

"I will stay focused and totally in control while at the store!"
Say this like you mean it.

Shopping day: _____
Groceries for the week:

Radiant Recipes

. . . .

Here's where the fun starts! In the next several chapters, you'll come to find that this way of eating not only makes you look gorgeous and feel amazing, but that it also tastes incredible! I encourage you to go through the recipes and choose the ones that appeal to you the most. Try to make the two weeks as enjoyable and delicious as you can—soon you'll find that achieving radiant health for life is easy, attainable, and scrumptious!

By now, you're probably familiar with the terms "green" and "blue," as explained on p. 7. However, here's a refresher course on all of the codes that appear after each recipe:

- **Green:** "Green" means go! These recipes are based on high-fiber whole foods, and are low in fat. They are the ideal foods to emphasize in your daily diet for optimum health. "Green" foods are what will comprise most of your menu on the two-week plan.

- **Blue:** "Blue" recipes tend to include higher-fat plant foods and/or natural sweeteners, making them something best eaten in moderation. You are allowed up to one serving of a "blue" recipe each day on the two-week plan.

- **GF:** This code means that the recipe is either already gluten-free, or that it can be made gluten-free with the suggested substitution(s).

- **SF:** For those who don't wish to consume soy products in any form, I've labeled the soy-free recipes as SF.

- **30 minutes or under:** This applies to recipes that can be made in—you guessed it—30 minutes or less! However, many other recipes without this tag are still incredibly easy to make. They may simply require soaking, marinating, dehydrating, or sprouting.

- ❄ : This symbol indicates that a recipe will freeze well.

Body-Loving Breakfasts

• •

The two-week plan is a great opportunity to rethink the way you begin each day. The best start is always the lemon water, as it will refresh and restore your system like nothing else! After that, you have some choices. As always, I recommend emphasizing nourishing things that you enjoy, all while following the guidelines of the plan.

Lemon Water

Fresh lemon water is *the* way to start the day! It wakes up your digestive system gently, and is cleansing and detoxifying. Lemon juice will also help to alkalinize your system, which assists your body in staying balanced and losing weight.

- ½-1 lemon (use one whole lemon if you can handle it!)
- 8-16 oz. warm or cold water (use filtered water or spring water if possible)

Cut the whole lemon into two halves. Using a citrus juicer (hand-held or electric), extract the lemon juice from the lemon. Add the desired amount of water to the lemon juice and drink. Feel the lemony love.

Serves 1/GF/SF/Green/30 Minutes or Under!

Alkalinizing? Say wha?

I often refer to foods (lemon water, for example) as alkalinizing. This means that they create a more alkaline (versus acidic) body. Having a highly alkaline body will help you to feel great, stay healthy, and lose weight with ease. Some specific examples of highly alkalinizing foods are vegetables, ginger, lemon, and mangoes.

Interestingly, many of the foods that are highly acid-forming are animal products, refined foods, coffee, and alcohol (the no-no's on this plan). In his book *Thrive*, Brendan Brazier (a vegan ironman triathlete) states that "an acidic body can lead to a plethora of health problems, including obesity and serious disease." [11]

However, on the Two-Week Wellness Solution, you don't have to keep track of which foods are which—you will naturally create a healthy, alkaline body just by eating the foods on this program! One less thing to worry about, right?

Veggie Vitality Juice

This vitalizing elixir will rev up your immune system, recharge your batteries, and make you feel like running a marathon! It can also serve as an optional replacement for the lemon water in the morning. I consider it to be two servings of vegetables.

- 2 medium carrots, washed well
- 1 large stalk of celery, washed well and bitter leaves removed
- 1 whole organic lemon, washed well (or ½ lemon if you aren't a huge fan of sour power) and cut into quarters
- 1 large handful parsley or kale (as much as you can handle, really)
- 1 small tomato, optional

Juice according to the manufacturer's guidelines for your juicer, then stir to mix. Fresh juices are best served right away as they begin to lose their vitamins quickly upon juicing. So drink up and feel fantabulous!

Serves 1/GF/SF/Green/30 Minutes or Under!

> If you have some "Immune-Boosting Tornado Tonic" (p. 87) on hand, try a squirt or two in this! It will even further increase the health benefits of this drink.

Green Radiance

This mega-nourishing drink will give your skin a glow, energize you, boost your immune system, and help put an end to unhealthy cravings. It will also detoxify your system and assist you with weight loss. I recommend drinking this every morning after your lemon water, before having your fruit. And although green drink mixes are readily available in health food stores, it's less expensive to make your own—plus, all of the ingredients in this drink have been specially selected for optimum health benefits.

One final note: The healthier you become, the more you'll enjoy the flavor of this drink. If you find it bitter at first, just give it time. Once your system has become cleansed by the two-week plan, you'll love it!

- 1½ cups dried nettle leaf (or ½ cup powdered nettles)
- 1½ cups dried peppermint leaf (or ½ cup powdered peppermint)
- ¼ cup barley grass powder
- ¼ cup spirulena powder
- 2 tablespoons dandelion leaf powder

1. If you're using non-powdered nettles and peppermint, you'll need to whir them in a food processor until powdered. This will take a minute, so be patient. Once powdered (or as powdered as they're gonna get), remove to a jar (or other container with a tight-fitting lid).

2. Add the barley grass, spirulena, and dandelion powders to the container. Cover tightly and shake well to mix. Store in a cool, dry place (or in the refrigerator) in an airtight container. This will remain fresh for at least a month.

3. To serve, stir 1-2 tablespoons into a glass of water. Alternatively, add it to a shake or smoothie if you prefer. Mix well and drink immediately. Feel radiant!

Makes 1¾ cups mix/GF/SF/Green/30 Minutes or Under! ❄

> I encourage you to harvest some of these wild greens yourself—nettles (wear gloves!), mint, and dandelion are readily available in the summer and can be easily dried. However, if you do need to buy the greens, Frontier Co-op sources high quality, organic ingredients. You can find them online at www.frontiercoop.com.

Immune-Boosting Tornado Tonic

This is incredibly easy to make and works like magic to stimulate your immune system and metabolism. I personally enjoy a teaspoon or two of this every morning (I drink it straight, like a "shot") after I've had my lemon water. However, for those who prefer milder foods, this can also be diluted in water or vegetable juice. Bring it on!

- 4 whole hot peppers (tabasco or cayenne peppers are ideal), chopped
- 5 large garlic cloves, chopped
- ¼ cup chopped ginger (unpeeled if organic)
- 2 tablespoons chopped turmeric root (you can substitute additional ginger if turmeric root is unavailable)
- 1 cup organic apple cider vinegar

1. Place all of the chopped items in a glass quart jar and cover with the apple cider vinegar. Close securely and shake well.

2. Place in the refrigerator for one month. During this marinating time, it's best to shake the mixture well every few days.

3. After the month is up, strain to remove all of the chopped items (they can be discarded or composted). Store the strained liquid in an airtight container in the refrigerator (or at room temperature in an amber bottle).

Makes about 1½ cups/GF/SF/Green

> *Tip:* When working with hot chilies, you should always wear gloves to keep the hot oils from burning your skin.

Frozen Bananas

Want to ensure your happy smoothie future? You've come to the right place.

- Ingredient: bananas (ripe or very ripe)

1. Peel the bananas and discard the peels (not onto the floor).
2. Break into 1 or 2-inch pieces and place in a plastic bag. Leave enough room so that the chunks can freeze individually. Seal the bag so that it's airtight.
3. Place in the freezer, laying the bag flat, so that the pieces can spread out and won't freeze together too much. After they've been frozen for 8-10 hours, they're ready. They will keep for several weeks or longer in the freezer. If at some point they do freeze together, simply thump the bag on the counter with feigned rage. They will separate out of fear.

Serves: the purpose/GF/SF/Green/30 minutes or under! ❄

Super Shake-A-Go-Go

For times when you want uber-nourishing sustenance on the go, this shake will deliver. This meal in a glass will energize you and give you a radiant complexion with its abundance of superfoods. Drink up and feel invincible!

- 1 cup **each**: frozen blueberries and soy yogurt (plain or vanilla)
- ½ cup nondairy milk
- 1 tablespoon **each**: ground flaxseed (flaxseed meal) and hemp protein powder (Nutiva is a good brand)
- One small handful of fresh kale, rinsed well
- *Optional:* 1 tablespoon agave nectar (omit if using sweetened milk)

Blend all of the ingredients in a blender until completely emulsified—this may take a minute! Drink up and purr.

Makes 1-2 Servings/GF/Green/30 Minutes or Under!

Beautiful Day Smoothie

This meal in a glass is such a mood booster! It contains beneficial enzymes from the pineapple juice, probiotics from the yogurt, and the highly nutritive benefits of mango and strawberries. It doesn't really matter which of your fruits are fresh or frozen, but for best results make sure at least one is frozen to ensure a thick consistency.

- 1 ripe mango, peeled and cut into chunks (you may use either one fresh mango or 1 cup frozen mango)
- 4 strawberries, fresh or frozen
- 1 cup soy yogurt, plain or vanilla
- ½ cup pineapple juice
- *Optional:* 1 tablespoon ground flax or hemp protein powder (or hemp seeds)

Blend all of the ingredients well. If necessary, add a little more pineapple juice (just enough to make your blender cooperate) and serve immediately. And, hey—you have yourself a beautiful day!

Makes 1-2 servings/GF/Green/30 Minutes or Under!

Berry Good Morning Shake

This shake is so rich and delicious that it's hard to believe it's so healthy and simple. Since berries are one of nature's best sources of antioxidants, vitamins, and fiber, you can drink up and feel fabulous!

- 2 frozen bananas (please see p. 88)
- 1½ cups berries (strawberries, blueberries, or raspberries), preferably frozen
- 1½ -2½ cups nondairy milk*
- 1 teaspoon vanilla extract

Place the frozen bananas, berries, 1½ cups of the milk, and the vanilla in a blender. Blend on low and then turn to high for several seconds to fully emulsify. Add more milk only if berry necessary.

Serves 2-3/GF/SF/Green/30 minutes or under! ❄

*The less liquid you add to a shake, the richer and thicker it will be. I give an estimated amount here, as it will depend on your blender and the size of the bananas as to how much milk you'll have to add. Simply start with the lesser amount given, and add a little more at a time until you have just enough liquid to blend with.

Sunshine Smoothie

This is like a beam of sunshine in a glass, and is pretty much my all-time favorite smoothie (in case you were wondering). It's simple, quick, and wonderfully nourishing! Mangoes are tri-doshic, which is an Ayurvedic term that basically means "great for all types of bodies."

- 1 frozen banana (please see p. 88)
- 1 mango, fresh or frozen*
- 1 cup orange-mango juice (or orange juice), the fresher the better

Place all of the ingredients in a blender and blend on low speed. After the ingredients begin to blend a bit, increase the speed to high until fully emulsified. Only add more juice (or water) if your blender can't do the trick with the amount specified. Drink up and bask.

Serves 2/GF/SF/Green/30 Minutes or Under! ❄

*Frozen mango works best, as it makes for a thick, creamy smoothie.

> To freeze mango, simply peel a ripe mango and cut it into 1-inch chunks, whittling down to the pod as best you can. Then, freeze in airtight plastic (leaving as much room as possible in between the chunks to avoid the annoying mango "ice block" situation). To save time, you can prepare several mangoes (and bananas) at once—plus, this will ensure a constant supply of this vitalizing smoothie!

Holiday Waffles (or Pancakes)

Just because you want to be healthy and trim doesn't mean you should deny yourself the good eats! This breakfast treat is high in fiber, low in fat, and absolutely delicious. For those of you who prefer pancakes, this recipe doubles just fine as a pancake recipe.

Flegg:
- 2 tablespoons ground flax (flaxseed meal)
- ¼ cup boiling water

Nog it Off:
- 1 cup vegan eggnog (or nondairy milk if vegan eggnog is unavailable)
- ¼ cup pureed squash or pumpkin

How Dry am I:
- 1 cup whole wheat pastry flour
- 1 teaspoon baking powder
- ⅛ teaspoon **each**: sea salt, cinnamon, and nutmeg

1. Place the ground flaxseed in a medium bowl, add the boiling water, and stir well. Allow it to sit undisturbed for at least 5 minutes so that it becomes gooey.

2. Stir the eggnog and squash into the gooey flegg mixture until well combined.

3. In a separate bowl, combine the dry ingredients, calmly ignoring the lame attempt at humor. Stir the dry mixture into the flax-squash mixture until well combined, but do not over-mix.

4. *If you're making waffles*: Use the batter according to the directions of your waffle maker. To ensure that your waffles come out easily, make sure the surface is hot enough and lightly sprayed with oil. Also, making smaller sized waffles usually ensures an easier process.

5. *If you're making pancakes*: Heat a large skillet over medium-high heat. If you don't have a truly nonstick pan, you may need to spray or lightly coat the skillet with oil (coconut or non-virgin olive oil being the best choices). When the pan is hot, drop the batter onto it to form a pancake-like shape. Do this again and again until you have several pancake-type formations on the skillet.

6. When they are very bubbly on top and browned on the bottom, flip over and cook the other side. When both sides are nicely browned, remove to a plate.

Repeat until all of the batter is gone. Serve hot, topped with applesauce or a drizzle of pure maple syrup or agave nectar.

Serves 2-3/SF/Blue/30 minutes or under! ❄

Waffle Lover's Tip:
When you have some time, make up a huge batch of waffles and freeze them (ideally in a single layer on a cookie sheet to prevent sticking). Once frozen, place them in an airtight bag and pop them back in the freezer. Then, anytime you want waffles you can simply heat them in your toaster, just like the pre-made, boxed variety!

Vegan Flax-Yogurt Superfood Pancakes

Once you taste these moist, delicious pancakes, you'll have a really hard time remembering how healthy they are! For an extra immune-boosting antioxidant kick, add the optional hemp and blueberries. Yum!

- 2 tablespoons ground flax (flaxseed meal)
- 3 tablespoons boiling water
- ½ cup vegan yogurt, plain or vanilla (I use Nancy's brand)
- 1 cup **each**: nondairy milk and whole wheat pastry flour
- ⅛ teaspoon sea salt
- ½ teaspoon **each**: baking soda and vanilla
- 1 teaspoon baking powder
- *Optional additions:* 1 tablespoon hemp protein powder and ½ cup blueberries

1. Place the flaxseed meal in a medium mixing bowl and pour the boiling water over it. Stir and allow it to sit for at least 5 minutes, or until gooey. Real gooey.

2. Stir in the yogurt and milk until well combined. Next, stir in the flour and salt until well combined. Finally, stir in the remaining ingredients until, yes, well combined. However, don't over-mix.

3. Heat a large skillet over medium-high heat and spray or coat lightly with oil (coconut or non-virgin olive are good choices). Once the skillet is hot, pour a little of the batter onto it, in shapes that resemble pancakes. Or little bunny heads.

4. Flip each pancake over when the underside is brown (it will be a little dry around the edges and bubbly on top). When both sides are gorgeously golden-browned, remove to a plate. Continue this process until all of your batter has been used up.

5. Serve with pure maple syrup or fresh berry syrup. Enjoy!

Serves 3/Blue/30 Minutes or Under!

> Flaxseed meal (ground flax) can either be purchased as such or made at home. To make your own, simply blend whole flaxseeds in a food processor or spice grinder until coarsely ground. This can take several minutes, especially in a food processor.

Apple Pie Amaranth Oatmeal

This simple concoction is warm, spicy, guilt-free comfort food. Plus, the amaranth adds a smattering of unique texture along with its amazing health benefits!

- 2 tablespoons dry amaranth
- 1¾ cups water

- ¾ cup **each**: rolled oats and finely diced apple (skins on if organic)
- ¼ cup raisins
- 2 tablespoons pure maple syrup (optional)
- 2 teaspoons vanilla extract
- ¾ teaspoon ground cinnamon
- ⅛ teaspoon **each:** sea salt and ground nutmeg

1. In a medium pot with a tight-fitting lid, place the amaranth and water over medium-high heat. Bring to a boil. Reduce the heat to low and simmer (still fully or partially covered) for 10 minutes.

2. Add the remaining ingredients and stir. Bring to a boil again over medium-high heat. Reduce heat to low and simmer (fully or partially covered) until all of the liquids have been absorbed (about 5-10 more minutes). Stir well and serve immediately. If desired, top with a little unsweetened nondairy milk.

Serves 2/GF (with gluten-free oats)/SF/Green/30 Minutes or Under! ❄

My recipe testers told me time and time again how much they loved this even better cold. I would have never thought of it!

Indian Spiced Supergrain Cereal

Here's a fabulously healthy way to start the day when you really need some nourishment. Plus, your home will smell divine while this is cooking!

- ¼ cup **each:** dry amaranth and dry quinoa, washed well and drained
- 1 cup water
- 5 whole cardamom pods (preferably green)
- ⅛ teaspoon ground ginger
- ½ teaspoon ground cinnamon
- ¼ teaspoon vanilla extract

- ¼ cup nondairy milk
- 1 tablespoon pure maple syrup
- *Optional:* 2 tablespoons raisins (or pitted, chopped dates)

1. In a small cooking pot, bring the amaranth, quinoa, water, cardamom, ginger, cinnamon, and vanilla to a boil over high heat, stirring well.

2. Reduce heat to low and simmer for about 10 minutes, or until the grains are tender and the liquid has been absorbed.

3. Remove the cardamom pods and add the remaining ingredients. Stir well and serve. Feel the power. Be it. Love it.

Serves 1-2/GF/SF/Green/30 minutes or under! ❄

Simple Sides

· · · · · · · · · · ·

These side dishes are simple, delicious, healthy, and easy to prepare. Many of them can also stand in as a main dish, especially the grain-based dishes. Enjoy, enjoy, enjoy!

Double Garlic Quinoa

Garlic likers, move on. There's nothing to see here. Garlic lovers, put on your seatbelts. This bad boy is quick, delicious, light, and super nourishing!

- 1 cup whole quinoa
- 2 cups water

- 6 large cloves garlic, peeled and thinly sliced
- 1 tablespoon extra-virgin olive oil

- 3 medium cloves garlic, minced or pressed
- 1 tablespoon **each:** minced fresh parsley and minced fresh basil (both very well packed)
- Sea salt and freshly ground pepper to taste

1. Rinse the quinoa in a fine mesh strainer and drain well. Place in a pot with the water. Cover and bring to a boil over medium-high heat. Reduce heat to low and simmer until all of the water has been absorbed, about 15 minutes.

2. While the quinoa is cooking, you can get all of the other ingredients ready. First, place the sliced garlic and olive oil in a small skillet over medium heat. Once it begins to sizzle, turn the heat down to medium-low and stir often. As soon as the garlic turns a beautiful shade of golden-brown, remove from heat. If you wait too long, the garlic will over-brown and become bitter.

3. Place the cooked quinoa in a large bowl and add the garlic-oil mixture. I like to use a rubber spatula to scrape all of the goodness out of the pan and into the quinoa, as it makes a difference in how the end product tastes.

4. Add all of the remaining ingredients, including the salt and pepper to taste. Toss gently with a spoon and serve. This will keep for several days, refrigerated in an airtight container. Buh-bye vampires!

Serves 3/GF/SF/Green/30 minutes or under!

Oven Roasted Cauliflower with Rosemary and Garlic

A woman recently told me that her husband now prefers this over steak! This deliciously addictive dish has also been referred to as "vegetable crack" by more than a few people.

- 2 teaspoons fresh rosemary leaf, stems removed and chopped
- 4 teaspoons olive oil, extra-virgin or regular
- 6 medium cloves garlic, minced or pressed
- ½ teaspoon sea salt (plus up to ⅛ teaspoon more if you like)
- ¼ teaspoon **each:** organic sugar (or sucanat) and ground black pepper
- ½ teaspoon balsamic vinegar
- 3½ cups chopped cauliflower (cut into bite sized pieces)

1. Preheat the oven to 400° F. Place everything but the cauliflower in a large bowl and stir to mix. Next, add the cauliflower and combine well with the seasonings using a rubber spatula. At this point you can allow the mixture to marinate for up to 24 hours (refrigerated in an airtight container) if you like.

2. Spread the mixture onto a large ungreased cookie sheet, using the rubber spatula to scrape all of the herbs and spices onto the cauliflower. Bake for about 15 minutes.

3. Turn the cauliflower over with a heat proof spatula and bake for another 10-15 minutes, or until lightly browned and very tender. Remove and serve. Feel impressed with yourself for as long as you like.

Serves 2/GF/SF/Green/30 minutes or under!

> This is a great side dish for Thanksgiving (or any special occasion) and can be prepared in advance. Simply toss all of the ingredients together and marinate overnight. Pop it into the oven half an hour before dinner and there you go! Simple elegance.

Kid's Choice Guacamole

Here's a creamy, non-spicy guacamole that is often first choice for adults as well! It's simple, quick, and tastes fresh and delightful. This guacamole is great served on a burrito, baked chimichanga, or any other fling that flaps your fancy.

- 1 avocado, ripe and ready
- 1 tablespoon **each:** fresh lime juice and minced fresh cilantro
- 1 medium clove garlic, minced or pressed
- ⅛ teaspoon sea salt

1. Remove the avocado flesh from its skin and place it in a bowl. Mash very well with a fork.

2. Stir in the lime juice, cilantro, garlic, and salt until very well combined. Although this is best served immediately, it will store for a day or two, refrigerated in an airtight container.

Serves 2-4/GF/SF/Blue/30 minutes or under!

Oven Glazed Tofu

I've been making this gooey, yummy baked tofu for well over a decade. It's nothin' fancy but makes for an irresistible and sustaining snack, sandwich filling, or sidekick.

Soy Important:
- 1 lb. extra firm (or firm) tofu

Marinade:
- 1 tablespoon oil (sesame, non-virgin olive, coconut, or sunflower)
- 1 teaspoon toasted (dark) sesame oil
- 2 tablespoons agave nectar or maple syrup
- 2 tablespoons **each:** tamari and cooking sherry or wine (it will cook off)

1. Slice the tofu horizontally into ¼-inch slabs in order to make 8 slices of tofu.

2. Press the tofu by laying it out in a single layer over paper towels. Place more paper towels on top and place a cutting board (or cookie sheet) over the top of it all. Next, place weights on the cutting board. You can use cans of beans, a gallon of water, a calm child, or a sleeping cat. Allow the tofu to press for as long as possible (up to 2 hours), but preferably at least 10 minutes.

3. Place the marinade ingredients in a large baking dish (such as a lasagna pan) and stir to combine. Place the pressed tofu into the pan in a single layer and coat all sides of the tofu with the marinade. Let marinate for at least 10 minutes (or up to an hour if you aren't experiencing a tofu-related emergency).

4. Preheat your oven to 400° F. Once the oven is hot, in goes the tofu.

5. Bake the tofu (uncovered) for about 20 minutes. Remove and turn each piece over using a heat proof spatula. Using a spoon (or tofurky baster), pour the extra sauce from the pan over the tofu.

6. Bake for another 20 minutes, or until the tofu is gorgeously well-browned and gooey. These should look very well done to ensure the maximum yum factor.

7. These will store, once cooled, in a covered container in the fridge for about five days. I think. I've never tested this theory, as they're just too yummy to have around that long in our house!

Serves 4/GF/Blue

Apricot-Glazed Asparagus

This I love. What a delicious way to get in your two cups of veggies at mealtime! Plus, it only takes about five minutes to make, start to finish.

- 2 cups chopped asparagus (trimmed and cut into 1-inch pieces)
- 1½ teaspoons **each:** water and tamari
- 2 tablespoons apricot fruit spread (all-fruit jam)
- 1 medium clove garlic, minced or pressed
- *Optional:* 1 teaspoon slivered or sliced almonds, toasted (dry toast in a pan over medium heat until lightly browned and aromatic)

1. In a medium skillet set to medium-high heat, sauté the asparagus in the water and tamari, stirring often. When the asparagus turns bright green and is crisp-tender, remove from heat. This should take well under 5 minutes.

2. Gently stir the apricot fruit spread and garlic into the asparagus until well mixed. Serve plain or topped with the almonds.

Serves 1/GF/Green/30 Minutes or Under!

Tip: To trim asparagus, hold the bottom of a stem with one hand and bend the top over with your other hand. Wherever the asparagus snaps is the natural separation between the inedible, tough base and the tender stem.

Zen Rice with Seaweed Gomasio

This is one of those dishes that I make frequently and really rely on. It is such the essence of lovely simplicity that I feel like I should be wearing a Zen monk's robe when I eat it! Both children and adults enjoy this dish, with or without the gomasio. Or robe.

- 1½ cups dry long grain brown rice (or brown basmati rice)
- 3 cups water
- 4 teaspoons (or more to taste) "Seaweed Gomasio" (p. 124)

- 8 teaspoons oil (coconut or olive)
- 4 teaspoons tamari, shoyu, or soy sauce
- 2 teaspoons nutritional yeast powder

1. Place the rice and water in a rice cooker, pressure cooker, or regular pot with a tight-fitting lid. Bring to a boil over high heat. Reduce heat to low and simmer until the water has been absorbed and the rice is tender. In a rice cooker or regular pot, this will take about 45 minutes. In a pressure cooker, this will take about 15 minutes or so once the top begins to shake and shimmy.

2. While the rice is cooking, make the gomasio. Set it aside.

3. Drizzle the cooked rice with the oil and tamari. Top with the nutritional yeast and gomasio and serve.

Serves 5-6/GF/Green ❄

Nutritional yeast. . .
Is a vitamin B-rich supplement that imparts a cheesy, nutty flavor to foods. It can be purchased in either flaked or powdered form—personally, I prefer the powder. You can find it in any health food store or in many supermarkets. Try it sprinkled over baked potatoes, popcorn, rice, or pasta for a yummy vitamin boost.

Quick and Healthy Herbed Garlic Bread

This bad boy has always been a hit with my weight loss clients as it satisfies the craving for garlic bread in a very healthy way.

- 4 slices sprouted or whole grain bread (such as Ezekiel 4:9 bread)
- 4 teaspoons olive oil (preferably extra-virgin)
- 4 medium cloves garlic, minced or pressed
- ½ teaspoon **each:** dried basil and dried oregano
- ⅛ teaspoon sea salt

1. Preheat the oven (or toaster oven) to 375° F.

2. Evenly drizzle each piece of bread with 1 teaspoon of oil. Spread each slice with one clove of garlic. Really distribute the oil and garlic evenly over the tops using a knife.

3. Sprinkle the spices and salt evenly over the bread slices. Place the bread directly on an oven rack for about 10-15 minutes, or until the garlic and bread begin to brown. Remove and serve immediately.

Serves 4/SF/Green/30 minutes or under! ❈

Cilantro-Lime Rice

I've had so many versions of this simple, tangy rice and loved them all. I especially like this version, as it's made with whole grain rice and lots of healthy, fresh ingredients! Enjoy.

- 1 cup long grain brown rice
- 2 cups water
- 2 tablespoons **each:** fresh lime juice and finely minced onion
- ¼ cup (packed) finely chopped fresh cilantro
- 1 medium-large clove garlic, minced or pressed
- 2 teaspoons oil (coconut, olive, or sunflower)
- ½ teaspoon sea salt (or less if you prefer)

1. Place the rice and water in a medium-sized covered pot and bring to a boil over medium-high heat. Reduce the heat to low and simmer (covered) until the rice is tender and all of the water is absorbed. This should take about 35-45 minutes.

2. Mix all of the remaining ingredients into the rice and stir well to combine. Serve immediately.

Serves 3/GF/SF/Green

Cranberry-Lime Confetti Quinoa

I've recently fallen in love with mixing a little red quinoa in with the regular tan-colored variety. It makes for a fun, visually appealing look (hence the "confetti"). Plus, it gives you the added nutritional benefits of red quinoa, while retaining the buttery taste of the regular variety.

- ½ cup dry quinoa, rinsed well and drained
- ¼ cup dry red quinoa, rinsed well and drained
- ½ cup orange juice
- 1 cup water

- ¼ cup **each:** minced green onions (or red onion, if you prefer a stronger onion flavor) and dried cranberries
- 2 tablespoons fresh lime juice
- 1 tablespoon agave nectar

- 2 tablespoons sliced or slivered almonds, toasted (toast over low heat in a dry pan until lightly browned)

1. Place the quinoas, orange juice, and water in a medium pot with a tight-fitting lid. Stir well. Cover and bring to a boil over high heat. Reduce heat to low and simmer (still covered) for 15 minutes, or until all of the liquids have been absorbed.

2. Meanwhile, place the remaining ingredients (all but the almonds) in a medium bowl. Once the quinoa is done, stir it into the bowl until well combined with the other ingredients. Serve topped with the almonds.

Serves 2-3/GF/SF/Green/30 Minutes or Under! ❄

> Quinoa is very nutritive, high in fiber, and contains loads of calcium and protein. Plus, it balances kapha. For those not familiar with Ayurvedic medicine, kapha is the body type that most easily tends toward weight gain. Eating kapha-balancing foods like quinoa is known to help keep the system in balance, which in turn promotes weight loss.

Springtime Bruschetta

For this appetizer, be sure to get the freshest, ripest tomatoes you can find, as it will make all the difference. Yum!

- 2 medium tomatoes
- 4 medium cloves garlic, minced or pressed
- ¾ teaspoon balsamic vinegar
- 10 medium basil leaves, finely chopped (or cut into thin ribbons)
- ¼ teaspoon sea salt
- 4 teaspoons olive oil (regular or extra-virgin)
- 4 slices sprouted grain (or whole grain) bread

1. Chop the tomatoes and place them in a strainer. Allow them to drain over a bowl (or the sink) for 5 minutes to remove the excess juices. You may wish to finger through them to assist this process.

2. Mix the garlic with the vinegar, basil, salt, and oil.

3. When the tomatoes have drained sufficiently, toss them with the basil mixture. Allow the tomato-basil mixture to marinate for about 15 minutes—or until the smell makes you a little crazy.

4. Grill or toast the bread and top with the mixture. Serve immediately.

Serves 4/SF/Green/30 minutes or under!

Quinoa Treasures Bowl

Nutritious, fresh, yummy, and easy to make. Now that's what I'm talking about!

Quinoa:
- 1 cup dry quinoa, rinsed and drained
- 2 cups water, preferably filtered

Treasures:
- The segments and minced zest of 1 large organic orange
- 2 tablespoons **each:** raisins and sliced kalamata olives
- 3-4 tablespoons minced red onion
- 1 teaspoon **each:** fresh lemon juice and extra-virgin olive oil
- ¼ teaspoon sea salt

Optional Flair: 2 tablespoons shelled pistachios, whole or crushed

1. Bring the quinoa and water to a boil in a covered pot. Reduce heat to low and simmer (partially covered) until all of the water has been absorbed—this will usually take about 15 minutes.

2. Toss the quinoa with all of the treasures and stir well to combine.

3. If desired, top with some pistachios. Serve immediately or refrigerate for up to two days.

Serves 4/SF/GF/Green/30 Minutes or Under!

Perfect Pinto Beans

These classic, delicious beans are perfect in Baked Chimichangas (p. 156), burritos, and tostadas.

- 1 cup dry pinto beans
- 2¼-3½ cups water
- 2-inch piece of kombu (p. 147)
- 2 bay leaves
- *Last Addition:* 1 teaspoon sea salt (or less if you prefer)

1. First, sort through the beans to remove any undesirable items such as stones, debris, bad beans, or nerd candy. Next, cover the pinto beans with plenty of water (about 4 cups or so). Allow them to soak overnight (or for 8-12 hours). However, if you don't have time to soak your beans, have no fear! You can still proceed confidently with this recipe.

2. Drain the soaked beans. Rinse them well. If you are using unsoaked beans, rinse them well and then drain them.

3. Place the beans in a pressure cooker (or pot with a tight-fitting lid). If you are using soaked beans, use the 2¼ cups of water. If you are using unsoaked beans, use the full 3½ cups of water. Place the kombu and bay leaves in the pot along with the water and beans.

4. Cover and bring to a boil over high heat. Reduce the heat to low and simmer until the beans are tender. For soaked beans, this takes about 45 minutes in a pressure cooker or 2 hours or more in a regular pot. For unsoaked beans, this will take about 70 minutes in a pressure cooker or 3 hours or more in a regular pot.

5. When your beans are tender, simply discard the kombu and bay leaves. As if they meant nothing to you. If you have too much liquid in the pot at this point, you may pour it out. Personally, I like to have a little bit of liquid left as much of it gets absorbed into the beans over time. Stir in the salt and there you have it!

Makes about 3 cups of beans/GF/SF/Green ❄

Scrumptious Salads

• • • • • • • • • • • • • • • •

Ah, salads. The elixir of freshness! This chapter should help solve the mystery of "How am I gonna eat all those veggies?" Plus, these salads are so delicious that you'll find yourself craving them instead of junk food—now isn't that something to look forward to?!

Almost Raw Asian Kale

This dish couldn't be simpler to prepare and is absolutely delicious! Kale is a nutritional powerhouse—it's insanely high in fiber, iron, chlorophyll, and immune-boosting properties. Dig in and feel the win!

- 6 cups kale (lightly packed), washed well and drained
- 2 tablespoons fresh lime juice
- 1 teaspoon toasted sesame oil
- 4 teaspoons agave nectar
- 1 tablespoon orange juice

- 5 medium cloves garlic, pressed or finely minced
- 1 tablespoon **each:** grated ginger and sesame seeds (raw or toasted)
- ¼ teaspoon sea salt

1. Remove the stems from the kale and chop the kale leaves into thin ribbons (or just finely chop if you prefer). Place in a large bowl.

2. Add the lime juice, sesame oil, agave nectar, and orange juice. Using your hands, stir well to combine. Continue to work the liquids into the kale with your hands—you are "massaging" the marinade into the kale. Once the kale turns a darker shade of green and is softened, you're done with the massage. Lights on, new-age music off.

3. Add the remaining ingredients to the kale mixture and stir well, using a spoon (or your hands). Once the mixture is thoroughly combined, it's done. This can either be served immediately or refrigerated in an airtight container for several days.

Serves 3/GF/SF/Green/30 Minutes or Under!

Mediterranean Chickpea Salad

This hearty salad also doubles as an entrée. Plus, it includes artichokes. How can you not love anything that includes artichokes?

- 1 teaspoon extra-virgin olive oil
- 1½ cups minced onion
- 2 stalks celery, thinly sliced or diced
- 8 medium-large cloves garlic, pressed or minced

- Two 15 oz. cans chickpeas, drained and rinsed (about 3 cups chickpeas)
- 1 cup artichoke hearts (not oil-packed)
- ½ cup marinated sun-dried tomatoes, julienne cut and drained
- 2 teaspoons extra-virgin olive oil
- ¼ cup liquid vegetable broth

- ¾ teaspoon sea salt
- ¼ cup fresh lemon juice
- Freshly ground black pepper to taste
- 2 teaspoons minced fresh rosemary (or 1 teaspoon dried)
- ½ teaspoon **each:** dried basil and dried oregano

- 4 cups baby greens or spinach, washed well and dried

1. In a large skillet set to medium-high heat, sauté the onion and celery in the 1 teaspoon of oil. Once the veggies are softened (about 5 minutes), add the garlic. Sauté for an additional minute.

2. Reduce the heat to medium-low and add the chickpeas, artichokes, sun-dried tomatoes, 2 teaspoons of olive oil, and vegetable broth. Stir well and cook for an additional minute.

3. Remove from heat and add the salt, lemon juice, pepper, rosemary, basil, and oregano. Gently stir well. If possible, allow the ingredients to marinate for about an hour before serving.

4. To serve, place the mixture on top of the baby greens (or spinach). This can be served warm, at room temperature, or cold. However, in the interest of maximum freshness, I don't recommend reheating it. Enjoy!

Serves 4/GF/SF/Green

Cucumber Dill Toss

This is the perfect solution to a summertime abundance of cucumbers and fresh dill. It's also fat-free, yummy, and highly nutritious. Cucumbers are renowned for their cleansing properties and dill is a wonderful aid to digestion.

- 2 medium-large cucumbers, very thinly sliced
- 1 medium red onion, very thinly sliced
- ¼ cup fresh dill (or more to taste), finely chopped
- 4 teaspoons agave nectar
- ½ cup apple cider vinegar
- ½ teaspoon sea salt

1. Place all of the ingredients in a large, airtight container and stir well to combine.

2. Refrigerate (tightly covered) for several hours or overnight to marry the flavors. You may want to occasionally take the container out and shake it a bit to make sure the marriage lasts. This will store for a week or more refrigerated in an airtight container.

Serves 4/GF/SF/Green

Five-Minute Five-Bean Salad

Here's a dish that you can toss together in no time (well, five minutes to be more specific) for a quick, satisfying main dish or side. It's also perfect for losing weight as it's fat-free, loaded with fiber, and low in calories. Plus, the beloved bean is very high in iron, minerals, and even Omega-3s—all nutrients that will help your body thrive.

- One 15 oz. can garbanzo beans (chickpeas)
- One 15 oz. can mixed beans (a blend of kidney beans, pinto beans, and black beans)*
- 1 cup thawed edamame (purchase it frozen and shelled for best results)

- ¾ cup minced scallions (green onions)
- ¼ cup apple cider vinegar
- 2 tablespoons **each:** agave nectar and fresh lime juice
- 1 teaspoon ground (dried) yellow mustard powder
- ¾ teaspoon sea salt (or less if you prefer)

1. Place the garbanzo beans, mixed beans, and edamame in a strainer (over a sink) and rinse well with water. Let drain while you're tossing the remaining items together.

2. Place all of the remaining ingredients in a medium-large bowl and stir well to combine.

3. Add the drained beans and edamame to the bowl and gently toss well so that all of the ingredients are thoroughly combined. Voila! Bean happiness at your fingertips. This dish will stay fresh for up to a week when refrigerated in an airtight container. On a final note, my recipe testers all told me that this dish is even better when allowed to marinate for several hours before serving. Enjoy!

Serves 4/GF/SF/Green/30 Minutes or Under!

*If you can't find organic canned mixed beans, you can simply substitute another type of beans such as kidney or pinto

Primavera Pasta Salad

This is a dish I made regularly for my weight loss clients many years ago—they loved the feeling of eating pasta without the guilt! This is far lower in fat than typical pasta salads and quite healthful due to the abundance of fresh veggies.

- 12 oz. package of organic whole grain pasta (fun shapes are encouraged)
- 1 cup liquid vegetable broth

Dressing:
- 3 tablespoons oil (preferably olive, flax, or hemp)
- 1½ tablespoons minced fresh rosemary
- ¼ cup plus 1 tablespoon umeboshi plum vinegar
- ½ cup red wine vinegar
- 6 medium cloves garlic, crushed or minced
- 3 tablespoons dried dill
- 1 tablespoon **each:** apple cider vinegar and poppy seeds

Veggie Love:
- 4 cups **each:** cherry (or grape) tomatoes and diced cucumber
- Medium red onion, minced
- Medium carrot, diced (about ½ cup)
- 2 medium celery stalks, trimmed and finely diced
- ⅓ cup kalamata olives, chopped

1. Cook the pasta according to the directions on its former home. Drain and gently toss with half of the veggie broth. Set aside.

2. Combine all of the dressing ingredients very well in a bowl using a whisk or fork. Stir the remaining vegetable broth into the dressing and set aside.

3. Prepare all of the veggies and place them in a ridiculously large bowl.

4. Add the noodles and dressing to the big bowl and combine well with the veggies. Use a gentle touch, especially if you're using gluten-free noodles. This dish is even better if it's allowed to marinate for an hour or more before serving.

Serves about 9 (at 2 cups per serving)/GF (with gluten-free pasta)/SF/ Green

Spinach Strawberry Salad

I've made this easy, elegant salad for more catering events than I can remember and it has never failed to garner rave reviews (and requests for the recipe!). If you have access to sorrel, it's a terrific addition. Simply substitute it for some of the spinach.

Delectable Dressing:
- 2 tablespoons **each**: oil (I use non-virgin olive), apple cider vinegar, and agave nectar
- 1 tablespoon **each:** sesame seeds, tamari, and orange juice
- ½ tablespoon poppy seeds
- ⅛ teaspoon paprika

Sweet Baby Salad:
- One 5 oz. bag of baby spinach, organic and pre-washed
- 1 pint strawberries, trimmed and thinly sliced
- *Topping:* ½ cup sliced almonds, toasted (dry toast in a pan over low heat until lightly browned)

1. Whisk the oil, vinegar, agave nectar, sesame seeds, tamari, orange juice, poppy seeds, and paprika together to make the dressing. Set aside.

2. Place the spinach (and sorrel, if using) and strawberries in a large bowl. Top with the dressing and toss to combine.

3. Top with the almonds just before serving. Warn your tummy about the overly intense fabulousness it is about to experience.

Serves about 4/GF/Green/30 minutes or under!

> *Note:* Be sure to use organic strawberries and spinach—it will make all the difference in the flavor and nutrition of this dish! Please see pages 61-62 for more details on organic foods.

Raw Catalonian Kale

The secret to tenderizing kale for use in raw dishes is to cut it finely and "massage" it with a marinade. However, this only takes minutes, and you'll be very pleased with the fresh, delectable, uber-nourishing results!

- 6 cups kale (lightly packed), washed well and drained
- 2 tablespoons fresh lemon juice
- 1 tablespoon **each:** extra-virgin olive oil and agave nectar

- 3-5 medium cloves garlic, pressed or finely minced (I use 5 cloves)
- ¼ cup raisins
- 8 Kalamata olives, pitted and quartered (or chopped)
- ¼ teaspoon sea salt

1. Remove the stems from the kale and chop the kale leaves into thin ribbons (or just finely chop if you prefer). Place in a large bowl.

2. Add the lemon juice, olive oil, and agave nectar to the kale. Next, roll up your sleeves—this is about to get interesting. Using your hands, toss well to combine. Continue to work the liquids into the kale with your hands—you are "massaging" the marinade into the kale. Once the kale turns a darker shade of green and is softened, it's ready for action.

3. Add the remaining ingredients to the kale mixture and stir well, using a spoon (or still using your hands if you're having too much fun). Once the mixture is thoroughly combined, it's good to go! This can either be served immediately or refrigerated in an airtight container for several days.

Serves 3/GF/SF/Green/30 Minutes or Under!

Spicy-Sweet Ginger Cabbage

This is one of my favorite ways to get in the two cups of veggies at lunchtime (heck, anytime!). Can you say "yummolicious?" However, this is a fairly spicy dish, so be prepared!

- ¼ cup thinly julienned* (not grated) fresh ginger
- ¼ cup plus 2 tablespoons fresh lime juice
- 3 tablespoons agave nectar
- ¾ teaspoon sea salt
- 6 cups (packed) very finely chopped (or grated) green cabbage
- ½-¾ teaspoon red chili flakes

1. Place the ginger in a very large mixing bowl. Add the lime juice, agave nectar, and salt. Stir well to combine.

2. Add the cabbage to the bowl and stir well. Using your hands, work the dressing into the cabbage. "Massaging" the cabbage will tenderize it without cooking—resulting in a raw, supremely nourishing and fresh dish. Once well combined, stir in the chili flakes with a large spoon.

3. Place in an airtight container and allow to marinate in the refrigerator for several hours (or overnight). Stir or shake every so often to assist the marinating process. Serve chilled. This will store for about seven days in the refrigerator.

Serves 3/GF/SF/Green

*Part of the appeal of this dish is that it contains tangible pieces of ginger. Hence, the anti-grating remark. To prepare the ginger, slice it first into thin rounds, and then slice each round into thin "sticks." Of course, if you have a mandolin, you can use that instead.

Indian Kuchumber Salad

This uber-fresh dish is tangy, addictive, and incredibly delicious. Oh, and by the way—it's good for you too!

- 1¾ cups diced cucumber (one medium cucumber), peel left on if organic
- ½ cup chopped tomato (or halved grape or cherry tomatoes)
- ¾ cup diced onion (red, white, or yellow)
- 2 tablespoons **each:** fresh lime juice and non-virgin olive oil
- ½ teaspoon **each:** sea salt and ground black pepper
- 3 tablespoons chopped fresh cilantro
- *Optional:* 1 teaspoon untoasted (raw) black sesame seeds

Gently toss all of the ingredients together until very well combined. Serve cold or at room temperature. This will store for several days, refrigerated in an airtight container.

Serves 4/GF/SF/Green/30 minutes or under!

Tess's Happy Salad

Everyone has a happy salad, and I invite you to discover yours. What kind of dressing do you love? What toppings make you smile? As long as you're using plant-based whole food ingredients, you too can create a scrumptious salad that will love you back. In the meantime, I hope you enjoy mine! It's quick, delicious, low-fat, vitamin-packed, and fulfills most of the day's vegetable requirement. Happiness!

- 2 teaspoons extra-virgin olive oil
- 2 tablespoons apple cider vinegar
- 1 teaspoon nutritional yeast (powdered)
- ¼ teaspoon ground black pepper
- ⅛ teaspoon sea salt
- 2 medium-large cloves garlic, pressed or minced

- 3 cups (lightly packed) Romaine or red leaf lettuce, chopped
- 1 cup artichoke hearts (water-packed, not marinated in oil)
- ¼ cup thinly sliced onion
- 4 kalamata olives, halved or chopped
- 6 grape or cherry tomatoes

1. In a medium-sized bowl, add the oil, vinegar, yeast, pepper, salt, and garlic. Stir well to combine.

2. Add the lettuce, artichokes, and onion. Toss well to combine. Serve garnished with the olives and tomatoes.

Serves 1/GF/SF/Green/30 Minutes or Under!

Sexy Seasonings, Saucy Sauces, and Divine Dressings

• • • • • • • • • • • • • • • •

In this chapter, you'll find all kinds of divinely delicious ways to flavor your foods without guilt. All of these recipes will also keep well, so I recommend finding your favorites and keeping them on hand so you'll have lots of yummy options for quick meals.

Sexy Seasonings

Saucy Sauces and Divine Dressings

Seaweed Gomasio

This tasty, nourishing condiment is perfect sprinkled over Zen Rice, quinoa, baked potatoes, beans, or salads. Let those sea minerals give you a glow!

- 1 cup brown (unhulled) sesame seeds
- ½ teaspoon **each:** dried garlic granules and dulse flakes
- 1 teaspoon sea salt
- ¼ teaspoon kelp powder
- ¼ sheet nori, torn into small pieces

Place all of the ingredients in a food processor and blend just until the sesame seeds are broken down and all of the seaweed is in small speckles—don't over-blend! Refrigerate in an airtight container (this will keep for months that way).

Makes about 1 cup of Gomasio/GF/SF/Green/30 minutes or under! ❄

Chicky Baby Seasoning

This all-purpose "chicken" flavoring puts an end to expensive store-bought seasonings—plus it's so much healthier! You can also use it to make a nice "chicken" broth (use one tablespoon of this mix per cup of water). It's especially delicious in soups, gravies, and rice pilaf—yum!

- 1 cup nutritional yeast powder
- 3 tablespoons **each:** dried onion granules and seasoned salt
- 2 teaspoons **each:** celery seed and dried garlic granules
- 2 tablespoons dried parsley flakes
- ½ teaspoon **each:** ground black pepper and white pepper
- 1 teaspoon **each:** lemon-pepper, sugar, dried dill, and dried rosemary

Combine all of the ingredients with a whisk or spoon until well mixed. Store in an airtight container out of direct sunlight. This will keep for several months.

Makes about 1½ cups/GF/SF/Green/30 minutes or under! ❄

Indian Seed and Spice Blend

These mixes make it very easy to throw an authentic Indian curry together in no time. Start by sautéing some of the seeds in a little hot coconut oil until they begin to pop. Then, add some of the spice blend and sauté another minute. Add some veggies and beans and you're good to go!

Indian Seeds Blend:
- 2 tablespoons **each:** black mustard seeds, cumin seeds, and sesame seeds

Indian Spice Blend:
- 1 tablespoon **each:** asafetida, red chili flakes, and dried turmeric
- 4 tablespoons **each:** cumin powder and coriander powder
- 1 teaspoon fenugreek
- 4 teaspoons amchur powder (dried mango), optional

1. Mix the seeds together and store them in a glass (or otherwise airtight) container. They will keep indefinitely.

2. Mix the spices together until they are well combined. Store them in a glass (or otherwise airtight) container. They will keep for several months, or indefinitely.

Makes about ⅓ cup of the seeds mix and ½ cup of the spice blend
GF/SF/Green/30 minutes or under! ❄

Thai Skinny Dipping Sauce

This yummy peanut sauce is always a big hit. It's perfect with fresh spring rolls, salads, Asian noodles, or stir-fries. Plus, you'll be so fit from eating all this delicious, healthy fare that you may want to go skinny dipping for real!

- ½ cup **each:** natural peanut butter and low-fat coconut milk
- ¼ cup **each**: fresh lime juice, agave nectar, tamari, and water
- ¼ cup **each**: fresh basil and fresh cilantro (well packed)
- 1 tablespoon chopped fresh ginger
- 4 cloves garlic, peeled
- *Optional and to taste:* ground cayenne or Sriracha sauce

Blend all of the ingredients in a blender until as smooth as possible (this may take a while). This will store in an airtight container, refrigerated, for up to ten days.

Makes about 2½ cups of sauce (about 20 servings at 2 tablespoons per serving) GF/Blue/30 minutes or under!

Fat-Free Maple Dijon Dressing

This dressing could not be simpler! It's perfect on salads, roasted veggies, potatoes, Brussels sprouts, quinoa, or just about anything else you can dream up!

- 2 tablespoons **each:** pure maple syrup and dijon mustard
- 1 tablespoon water
- ½ teaspoon poppy seeds

Whisk or stir all of the ingredients together and serve. This will last, refrigerated in an airtight container, for a month or more.

Serves 2/GF/SF/Green/30 Minutes or Under! ❄

Mango Habanero Sauce

Oh sweet elixir of heat. How I love this sauce! It's perfection on top of black beans, burritos, baked chimichangas, quesadillas, or tempeh. However, it's very spicy, so you may want to start with just a few drops. Enjoy!

- ½-1 habanero pepper (use a whole pepper for maximum heat)
- 2 ripe mangoes, peeled
- ½ teaspoon sea salt
- 1 tablespoon agave nectar or organic sugar
- ¼ cup fresh lime juice

1. Preheat your oven to broil (the highest setting). Wash the habanero.

2. Place the habanero under the broiler and allow it to cook until it's well roasted. You'll want to turn it over mid-way so that both sides become browned. There isn't an exact amount of time as ovens vary—just check often during this process as you don't want it to burn. Once the habanero is nicely browned on both sides, remove it and turn the oven off.

3. Cut the habanero in half. Remove the seeds, inner white portion, and stem.

4. In a food processor or blender (or using a hand blender), blend the roasted habaneros with all of the remaining ingredients until very smooth. Hot velvet is what you're going for here. This will keep for 2 weeks (or longer) in an airtight container (preferably glass), refrigerated.

Makes 2 cups of sauce (about 16 servings)
GF/SF/Green/30 Minutes or Under! ❋

> Get out the gloves—you'll want to wear them while handling the habaneros, as they're the hottest pepper known to humankind. I keep some cheap plastic gloves under my kitchen sink for just this purpose.

Light Balsamic Dressing

Balsamic vinegar is ideal for low-fat dressings as its full, rich flavor makes extra oil superfluous. Plus, this yummy dressing is ready to go in under five minutes! Win.

- 1 tablespoon **each:** orange juice and olive oil
- ¼ cup plus 2 tablespoons balsamic vinegar
- 2 tablespoons pure maple syrup (or agave nectar)
- ½ teaspoon poppy seeds
- ¼ teaspoon **each:** sea salt and ground black pepper
- 1 teaspoon tamari, shoyu, or soy sauce

Whisk or stir all of the ingredients together. This will keep in the fridge for several weeks or more. This is best if brought to room temperature before serving.

Makes ½ cup of dressing (4 servings)/GF/Green/30 minutes or under!

Light Ginger-Miso Dressing

This cleansing, ultra-nourishing dressing is just delicious over green salads, shredded cabbage, or cold soba noodles.

- 2 tablespoons mellow white miso (do not use dark miso here)
- ½ cup orange juice (the fresher the better)
- 1 tablespoon grated fresh ginger
- 2 tablespoons toasted (dark) sesame oil
- ¼ cup **each:** fresh lemon juice and agave nectar (or organic sugar)
- 2 tablespoons tamari, shoyu, or soy sauce

1. Whisk the miso with the orange juice until smooth.

2. Add the remaining ingredients and stir or whisk well to combine. This will store for two weeks or more in an airtight container in the fridge.

Makes 1 cup of dressing (8 servings)/GF/Green/30 minutes or under!

Healthy Snacks and Starters

· ·

After reading this chapter, you may wonder if I need to join a support group for spring roll addicts. The answer is simple—yes, I do. However, in my defense, fresh spring rolls are pretty much perfect. They're snacky, delicious, crunchy, satisfying, and filled with all manner of body-nourishing goodness. Of course, there are other recipes in this chapter too. Here you'll find new ideas for snacks as well as tasty complements to any meal—all meant for your enjoyment and wellness. So here's hoping these recipes will inspire you to enjoy every minute of your journey to optimum health!

Boostcorn

This is a simple popcorn snack that I make often as it's filling, low in fat, and chock-full of health supporting ingredients. In particular, coconut oil and chilies are highly renowned for boosting the metabolism and revving up the immune system. Plus, nutritional yeast is rich in B-vitamins and high-fiber popcorn is the perfect food for losing weight and staying energized.

- 1 tablespoon coconut oil
- ⅓ cup popcorn kernels

- ½ teaspoon **each:** garlic granules and onion granules
- 2 teaspoons nutritional yeast powder
- *To taste:* hot sauce of your choice and sea salt

1. Place a heavy pot with a tight-fitting lid over medium-high heat. Add the coconut oil and the popcorn.

2. To prevent the popcorn from burning, you'll want to shake the pot frequently (be sure to hold onto the lid with hot pads while you shake it). This will distribute the oil and keep the popcorn kernels from sticking to the bottom. Continue to cook until the popping slows down to 1-2 seconds in between pops. Remove from heat.

3. Empty the popped corn into a large bowl. Sprinkle with the seasonings and add the hot sauce to taste. I like to stir using a rubber spatula so that all of the seasonings are properly distributed. Pop in your favorite movie and you're good to go!

Serves 1-2/GF/SF/Green/30 Minutes or Under!

> Garlic and onion granules are the same as granulated garlic and onion. Instead of powdered onion and garlic, I prefer to use the granules—they're much more flavorful and don't have a bitter aftertaste. You can find them in most supermarkets and health food stores.

Spicy Sweet Potato Fries

French fries specially formulated for weight loss? Oh yeah. These so-called fries deliver the flavor while speeding up your weight loss with high-fiber, low-fat yumminess. Incidentally, coconut oil is the best oil for weight loss as it's high in medium-chain fatty acids (the kind that aren't stored as fat). Plus, the cayenne will boost your metabolism as well. Enjoy the guilt-free goodness!

- One small (5 oz.) orange-fleshed sweet potato (often labeled as a yam), unpeeled
- 1 teaspoon **each:** fresh lime juice and melted coconut oil
- ½ teaspoon organic sugar
- ¼ teaspoon sea salt
- ⅛ teaspoon ground turmeric
- A few dashes ground cayenne powder (up to ⅛ teaspoon if you love heat!)

1. Preheat your oven to 375° F. Wash the sweet potato well and cut it into ¼-inch thick slabs. Next, cut each slab into sticks. What you're going for here are relatively thin French fry shapes. You should end up with 1½ cups of sweet potato sticks.

2. In a small bowl, toss the sweet potato sticks with all of the remaining ingredients. I use a rubber spatula to make sure everything gets thoroughly mixed together.

3. To bake, you'll want to either have a very good nonstick pan or a silpat liner, as the low-fat nature of these fries makes them prone to sticking. Spread them out on your pan in a single layer, making sure they aren't overlapping. Bake for 15 minutes, then remove and turn the fries over so that they cook evenly. Bake for another 15 minutes, then check for doneness. They are done when they're tender and lightly browned. Remove and serve immediately.

Makes 1 serving/GF/SF/Green

Edamame Spring Rolls with Orange-Miso Sauce

These babies contain a plethora of extremely health-boosting ingredients. Miso is a powerful detoxifying agent, while the ginger and fresh veggies boost the immune system. Edamame is a high-fiber whole food that is often well tolerated by those otherwise avoiding soy. I recommend buying frozen, pre-shelled edamame—so user-friendly!

- 1 "nest" (1.76 oz.) bean thread noodles
- 8 spring roll wraps (rice paper)

Orange-Miso Sauce:
- 3 tablespoons tahini
- ½ cup orange juice
- 2 tablespoons **each:** agave nectar, tamari, grated ginger, toasted sesame oil, mellow white miso, and fresh lime juice

Fresh Fillings:
- 1 cup **each**: shelled edamame (thawed), chopped cilantro, chopped Romaine lettuce, and grated carrot
- 4 green onions, trimmed and sliced in half to form eight 3-inch pieces

Tasty Toasty Topping:
- 1 tablespoon toasted sesame seeds (toasted in a dry skillet over low heat until lightly browned)

1. Place all of the "Orange-Miso Sauce" ingredients in a blender and blend until smooth. Set aside.

2. Next, prepare the bean threads according to the instructions on their package. Rinse them in a strainer under cold water and cut them a few times so that they aren't quite as long. I usually keep these in the strainer the entire time I'm preparing the spring rolls, as it's important to use well drained noodles.

3. Prepare all of your "Fresh Fillings" and set them aside.

4. Find a pan or bowl large enough to put the rice paper wrappers in. Fill it two inches high with lukewarm or cool water. Place a sheet of rice paper in the water, making sure that it's covered entirely with the water. In a minute or less, it should soft. Don't over-soak the wrapper, or it will tear more easily.

5. Remove the wrapper and allow any excess water to drip off of it. Lay it flat on a clean surface. Place a little of each filling ingredient (bean threads, edamame, cilantro, lettuce, carrots, and a scallion segment) in the middle of the wrapper. Don't overfill, or it will be tricky to roll. Roll the bottom of the rice paper wrapper up and over the fillings. Next, fold the left and right sides in—if you can maintain parallel lines, it will produce a more even looking wrap. Finally, finish rolling it all of the way up. The rice paper will self-seal, so just set the spring roll aside and repeat this process until all of your fillings are used up.

6. Top each spring roll with some of the toasted sesame seeds. They should stick to the rice paper without any help, but you can always sprinkle a little water on top of your spring rolls to assist the process if necessary. Serve with the "Orange-Miso Sauce" and enjoy the yummy health boost!

Makes 8 spring rolls (serves 4-8)/GF/Green/30 Minutes or Under!

Did you know?

Miso is an amazing superfood! It's highly detoxifying, cleansing, and immune-boosting. Just the thing to prevent or cure illnesses, miso is delicious and soothing as well. Be sure to never boil it, however, as that will destroy miso's nutrients. Dark miso is the most nutritious type of miso, although it's also less versatile than the light varieties—I tend to use dark miso just for soups. However, I use light, mellow white miso in everything from soups to salad dressings to sauces to sandwich spreads. Yum!

Rawsome Energy Cookies

These cookies, made using only whole foods, are my new favorite snack on the go. Their nutrient-rich ingredients will give you loads of energy, glowing health, and a radiant complexion! There are four different kinds of cookies here, so have fun finding your favorite—or do some experimenting of your own!

Note: Be sure to use regular pearled barley (the same kind you'd make soup from), not barley sprouts, for best results. Enjoy!

Gooey Cinnamon-Raisin
- ½ cup **each:** dry pearled barley, raisins, and pitted dates
- ¼ cup **each:** raw walnuts and raw pecans
- 1½ teaspoons ground cinnamon
- ½ teaspoon sea salt

Zesty Lemon
- ½ cup **each:** dry pearled barley, raw almonds, and pitted dates
- ¼ cup raisins (omit if you prefer a less sweet, stronger lemon flavor)
- 3 tablespoons fresh lemon juice
- 1 tablespoon (packed) minced lemon zest
- ½ teaspoon sea salt

Blueberry Lemon Lovelies
- ½ cup **each:** dry pearled barley, raw pecans, and raisins
- 2 tablespoons fresh lemon juice
- 1 tablespoon (packed) minced lemon zest
- ½ teaspoon sea salt
- *Add last:* ¼ cup dried blueberries

Cranberry-Orange Spice
- ½ cup **each:** dry pearled barley, raw almonds, and pitted dates
- 2 tablespoons fresh orange juice
- 2 teaspoons (packed) minced orange zest
- ½ teaspoon sea salt
- ⅛ teaspoon ground nutmeg
- *Add last:* ½ cup dried cranberries

1. *To prepare the barley for one batch of cookies:* Place the ½ cup of barley in a sprouting jar (or quart-sized glass jar) and cover well with water. Let sit for 8 hours, or overnight. Pour off the water, then rinse with water again. Drain and place upside-down in a bowl at a 45° angle for another 8-12 hours. Continue to rinse and drain the barley every morning and evening (still storing it upside-down at a 45° angle). After about two days, the barley will be tender, yet still a bit chewy—this means it's done (it won't actually look sprouted). Once the barley is ready, it's important to stop "sprouting" it and use it right away (or refrigerate for up to two days if necessary). Rinse and drain once again, for old time's sake.

2. In a food processor, blend the barley well. Add the remaining ingredients for whichever batch of cookies you've chosen and blend thoroughly.

Note: If you're making "Blueberry Lemon Lovelies" or "Cranberry-Orange Spice" cookies, you'll want the blueberries and cranberries to remain whole. To do this, blend all of the other ingredients until well mixed. Then, stir or lightly pulse in the berries, just until well mixed.

3. To form the cookies, roll one tablespoon of the mixture into a ball. Repeat 19 times. At this point, you can either dry the cookies in a food dehydrator (recommended) or simply serve as is. If you're going to use a food dehydrator, press the cookies until they're semi-flat and place them in the dehydrator. Allow them to dry at 105° F for about 12 hours. When they're done, they should be chewy and relatively soft (not brittle). Once dehydrated, these happy babies will store for several weeks in an airtight container at room temperature. If not dehydrated, they will keep for several days, refrigerated in an airtight container.

Each batch makes 20 cookies (2-3 cookies per serving)/SF/Green ❋

> Inexpensive sprouting set-ups are available online if you can't find one at your local health food store. All you need is a quart-sized glass jar and a lid with air holes.

> I'll never forget how much fun I had creating this recipe! My 6-year-old and her friend Lili helped me stir, shape, and taste-test all of the cookies. Wide-eyed and enthusiastically asking for more, they affirmed that children really do love healthy food!

Shiitake-Basil Spring Rolls

Fresh spring rolls—my raison d'être. Plus, there's even more reason to go on living with *these* spring rolls, as they're simultaneously satisfying, yummy, uber-nourishing, and light! Chow down and feel gooooood.

- ½ cup of the "Thai Skinny Dipping Sauce" (p. 126)
- 1 "nest" (1.76 oz.) bean thread noodles
- 6 spring roll wraps (rice paper)

Good Shiit:
- 3 cups sliced shiitake mushroom caps, fresh or frozen
- 1 tablespoon tamari
- 1 teaspoon toasted sesame oil
- 3 large garlic cloves, minced or pressed

Getting Fresh:
- ½ cup (chopped) **each:** fresh basil, fresh cilantro, and Romaine lettuce
- 1 large carrot, julienne cut or grated
- 3 scallions (green onions), trimmed and sliced in half to form six 3-inch pieces

Tasty Topping:
- 2 teaspoons toasted sesame seeds (toasted in a dry skillet over low heat until lightly browned)

1. First, you'll want to make the "Thai Skinny Dipping Sauce" if you haven't already. Next, prepare the bean threads according to the instructions on their package. Rinse them in a strainer under cold water and cut them a few times so that they aren't quite as long. I usually keep these in the strainer the entire time I'm preparing the spring rolls, as it's important to use well drained noodles.

2. Heat a large skillet over medium-high heat. Add the shiitakes, tamari, sesame oil, and garlic. Sauté, stirring often, for 5 minutes, or until the mushrooms are dark brown and tender. Set aside.

3. Prepare all of your "Getting Fresh" filling ingredients and set them aside.

4. Find a pan or bowl large enough to put the rice paper wrappers in. Fill it two inches high with lukewarm or cool water. Place a sheet of rice paper in the water, making sure that it's covered entirely with the water. It should be soft in less than

a minute—don't over-soak the wrapper, or it will tear more easily.

5. Remove the wrapper and allow any excess water to drip off of it. Lay it flat on a clean surface. Place a little of each filling ingredient (including the bean threads, shiitakes, and "Getting Fresh" items) in the middle of the wrapper. Don't overfill, or it will be tricky to roll. Roll the bottom of the rice paper wrapper up and over the fillings. Next, fold the left and right sides in—if you can maintain parallel lines, it will produce a more even looking wrap. Finally, finish rolling it all of the way up. The rice paper will self-seal, so just set the spring roll aside and repeat this process until all of your fillings are used up.

6. Top each spring roll with some of the toasted sesame seeds. Serve with the sauce and savor the health-supporting flavors!

Makes 6 spring rolls/GF/Green

> *Tip:* When using organic ginger root, there is no need to peel it. Simply wash it well and then grate, mince, or julienne as desired. In fact, many of ginger's nutrients are located just under the skin, making unpeeled ginger an even healthier choice. Ginger is wonderfully cleansing, anti-inflammatory, immune-boosting, and stimulating. Ginger—pure proof that life is good!

Summer Rolls with Chili-Lime Sauce

Yum. Enough said.

- 12 spring roll wrappers (rice paper)

Chili-Lime Sauce:
- ¼ cup **each:** spicy Thai chili sauce (I use Thai Kitchen brand) and tamari
- ⅓ cup fresh lime juice
- 8 large cloves garlic, minced or pressed
- 4-5 teaspoons grated fresh ginger

Bean Threads:
- 1 nest (1.76 oz.)
- *Optional:* 1 teaspoon toasted sesame oil

Fillin' The Love:
- 6 scallions (green onions), trimmed and sliced in half to make twelve 3-inch segments
- ½ cup crushed peanuts
- ¾ cup **each:** julienned carrots, fresh mint, and chopped fresh cilantro
- 12 mango spears (about three inches in length and ¼-inch in diameter)
- 12 cucumber spears (about three inches in length and ¼-inch in diameter)

Over the Top:
- 4 teaspoons toasted black or regular sesame seeds (toasted in a dry skillet over low heat until lightly browned)

1. Combine all of the "Chili-Lime Sauce" ingredients in a bowl. Stir and set aside.

2. Cook the bean threads according to the directions on their package. Drain and cut them into smaller segments. Toss with the sesame oil (if this is what you deeply desire) and set aside.

3. Prepare all of the filling items and set them aside. Don't forget the love.

4. Find a pan or bowl large enough to put the rice paper wrappers in. Fill it two inches high with lukewarm or cool water. Place a sheet of rice paper in the water, making sure that it's covered entirely with the water. It should be soft in less than a minute—don't over-soak the wrapper, or it will tear more easily.

5. Remove the wrapper and allow any excess water to drip off of it. Lay it flat on a clean surface. Place a little of each filling ingredient (including the bean threads) in the middle of the wrapper. Don't overfill, or it will be tricky to roll. Roll the bottom of the rice paper wrapper up and over the fillings. Next, fold the left and right sides in—if you can maintain parallel lines, it will produce a more even looking wrap. Finally, finish rolling it all of the way up. The rice paper will self-seal, so just set the spring roll aside and repeat this process until all of your fillings are used up.

6. Top with some sesame seeds and serve with the dipping sauce. Enjoy!

Makes 12 summer rolls/GF/Green

For those who are new to the mango-cutting scene...
A word of warning: Cutting a mango is a messy, unruly job and no one gets out alive. However, you can minimize the heartache by proceeding as follows: Peel the mango (over a plate—it's juicy!) and then cut it into "slabs." Work around the pod (pit) as best you can, which won't be all that great. Next, cut the slabs into ½-inch sticks. Finally, suck on the pod if you're the kind of person who likes to savor as much flavor as you can, while you can.
p.s. Be sure to have some dental floss handy.

Vietnamese Spring Rolls

I have a special place in my heart for Vietnamese spring rolls—they were my first introduction to fresh spring rolls, many moons ago, in a small Vietnamese restaurant. Although my taste buds weren't sold on them at first, my body knew better. I began to crave them like crazy only days after trying them. The sprouts, ginger, garlic, and greens make my system sing for joy!

- ½ lb. firm tofu
- 4 teaspoons tamari, shoyu, or soy sauce
- ¾ teaspoon **each:** dried garlic granules and dried onion granules
- 2 teaspoons toasted sesame oil

Simple Sauce:
- ¼ cup plus 2 tablespoons **each:** hoisin sauce (available in most supermarkets and Asian markets) and water

Fillin' Good:
- 12 (yeah, you heard me!) medium cloves garlic, pressed or minced
- 2 tablespoons finely grated fresh ginger (or more if you prefer)
- 1 cup bean sprouts (fresh), lightly packed
- ¾ cup (packed) chopped cilantro
- ¾ cup (lightly packed) chopped Romaine (or red leaf) lettuce
- 6 green onions, trimmed and sliced in half to form twelve 3-inch pieces

Oh Sheet:
- 12 spring roll skins (rice paper sheets)

1. Cut the tofu into four slabs and press them well with paper towels to remove the excess water. Cut each slab into three long sticks. You should now have twelve tofu sticks. Place the tofu on a plate and coat all sides with the tamari, garlic granules, and onion granules. Allow them to marinate for a few minutes, then place in a medium skillet in the sesame oil. Pan-fry over medium-high heat until the tofu is evenly browned (about 2-4 minutes on both sides). Set aside.

2. Combine the hoisin sauce and water until well mixed. Set aside.

3. Prepare all of the fillings so that everything you need is now ready to go.

4. Find a pan or bowl large enough to put the rice paper wrappers in. Fill it two inches high with lukewarm or cool water. Place a sheet of rice paper in the water,

making sure that it is covered entirely with the water. In a minute or less, it should be soft. Don't over-soak the wrapper, or it will tear more easily.

5. Remove the wrapper and allow any excess water to drip off of it. Lay it flat on a clean surface. Place a little of each filling item in the middle of the wrapper. Don't overfill, or it will become a salad. A delicious, messy salad.

6. Roll the bottom of the rice paper wrapper up and over the fillings. Next, fold the left and right sides in—if you can maintain parallel lines, it will produce a more even looking wrap. Finally, finish rolling it all of the way up. The rice paper will self-seal, so just set the spring roll aside and repeat this process until all of your fillings are used up. Serve with the hoisin sauce.

Makes 12 spring rolls (serves 6)/GF/Green

Spring Roll Lover's Tips:

♥ I always keep fresh spring roll fillings on hand in the fridge (in individual airtight containers). That way, I can make spring rolls anytime—fast and fresh!

♥ If you do end up making more spring rolls than you can eat immediately, they can be successfully stored—with the help of this trick: Wrap each spring roll in a damp paper towel and refrigerate in an airtight container. They will keep for several days this way.

Fresh Cukocado Spring Rolls

These freshlings make for a great mini-meal or a sustaining snack.

Tangy Lime Dipping Sauce:
- Juice of 1 lime
- 2 tablespoons **each:** tamari and spicy Thai chili sauce (I use Thai Kitchen brand)
- 2 teaspoons agave nectar

Fillings (Nothing but Fillings):
- 1 avocado, peeled and cut into spears
- 1 cucumber, peeled and cut into 3-inch spears
- 3 green onions, trimmed and cut in half to make six 3-inch segments
- ¾ cup **each:** chopped cilantro and chopped red leaf lettuce
- 1 lime, cut into wedges

Wrap It Up Already:
- 6 rice paper wrappers (spring roll skins)

1. Prepare the sauce by stirring the "Tangy Lime Dipping Sauce" ingredients together. Set aside.

2. Prepare all of the fillings and set aside.

3. Find a pan or bowl large enough to put the rice paper wrappers in. Fill it two inches high with lukewarm or cool water. Place a sheet of rice paper in the water, making sure that it is covered entirely with the water. In a minute or so, it should be soft. Don't over-soak the wrapper, or it will tear more easily.

4. When the wrapper is soft, place it on a clean, dry surface.

5. Place a little of each filling (everything but the lime) in the center of the wrapper. Squeeze a lime wedge over the top to juice things up a little.

6. Fold the bottom of the rice paper up and over the fillings. Then, fold in the sides (maintaining parallel edges). Finally, finish rolling it all of the way up until you have a beautiful, new spring roll infant. It will self-seal so just set it aside.

7. Repeat with the remaining five wrappers. Serve with the dipping sauce. Yum!

Makes 6 spring rolls/GF/Green/30 minutes or under!

Indian Snacky Taters

This snack is very quick and easy to make—plus, it satisfies the urge for fried potatoes in a low-fat, healthy way. Even if you don't have the "Indian Spice Blend" on hand, this dish will still come together in under fifteen minutes (although you do have to have a cooked, cooled potato on hand). You can also have fun experimenting with other flavor combinations—try Cajun, Mexican, Greek, or Moroccan spices for some alternative snacky fun.

- 1 medium potato, baked and cooled
- 1 teaspoon **each:** coconut oil and "Indian Spice Blend" (p. 125)
- ¼ teaspoon granulated garlic (garlic granules)
- Sea salt to taste
- *Optional for dipping:* chutney or ketchup

1. If you haven't made the "Indian Spice Blend" yet, now is the time.

2. Preheat a medium-large skillet over medium heat and add the coconut oil.

3. Slice the potato into ¼-inch rounds and place on a plate. Sprinkle each side of the potato evenly with the spice blend and garlic granules. Place in a single layer on the skillet and cook for 2-3 minutes, or until the undersides are brown.

4. Flip each slice over and cook another 2-3 minutes, or until both sides are browned. Remove and season with sea salt to taste. Serve with chutney or ketchup and get your snack on!

Serves 1/GF/SF/Green
30 Minutes or Under! (if you have cooked potatoes on hand) ❄

To plan ahead for this dish. . .
Toss a few potatoes in the oven and bake them when you're already using the oven. The pre-baked potatoes will keep for several days in the fridge. . . as they eagerly await their snacky fate.

Slimming Soups

· · · · · · · · · · · ·

Soups are hands-down one of the best weight-loss foods ever. The good ones fill you up, not out, and pack in loads of fiber and nutrients. For more choices in the world of soup, you can also refer to **Radiant Health, Inner Wealth** or the list of "green" packaged soups on p. 185.

Get Skinny Soup

This is the perfect soup for trimming down as it's very low in fat and calories, extremely high in fiber, and oddly satisfying!

- 1 medium carrot, thinly sliced
- 1 medium stalk of celery, thinly sliced
- ¾ cup finely chopped onion (one small-medium sized onion)
- 1 tablespoon extra-virgin olive oil
- 7 cups water, preferably filtered
- 2 cups chopped green cabbage
- 1 cup dry lentils (green or brown), rinsed well and sorted
- One 14.5 oz. can diced tomatoes with garlic and onions (juice and all)
- 1½ teaspoons **each:** dried oregano and agave nectar
- 2 bay leaves
- 3-inch piece kombu (p. 147)

- 1 teaspoon sea salt
- Lots of freshly ground black pepper, to taste (I use about ¾ teaspoon)
- ½ teaspoon balsamic vinegar
- 3-5 medium cloves garlic, pressed or minced
- *Garnish:* 16 basil leaves, cut into thin ribbons

1. In a large soup pot, sauté the carrot, celery, and onion in the oil over medium-high heat for about 5 minutes, or until the veggies begin to soften.

2. Add the water, cabbage, lentils, tomatoes, oregano, agave, bay leaves, and kombu. Bring to a boil over high heat. Reduce heat to low and simmer, partially covered, until the lentils are soft. This will take about an hour.

3. Once the lentils are tender, remove the bay leaves and kombu. Stir in the salt, pepper, vinegar, and garlic. Ladle into bowls and garnish with the basil. This will store refrigerated for up to ten days.

Makes about 6 servings/GF/SF/Green ❄

Although it's rare to find pebbles, dirt, and other outlaws in your dry beans and lentils, it's still a good idea to rinse and sort them. It can actually be a very enjoyable ritual as well. Allow yourself to slow down, breathe, and savor the feeling of running your fingers through the dry legumes.

Lickety Split Pea Soup

Nothing fancy here—just down-home healthy, comforting, slurpy goodness. This soup is also a personal favorite as it only involves about five minutes of actual work and provides daily nourishment for the rest of the week. Hard to beat that!

Into the Big Pot:
- 1 scant cup green split peas (2 tablespoons shy of a full cup), rinsed
- 4½ cups water
- 2 bay leaves
- 4-inch segment kombu (please see tip at the bottom of this page)
- 3 tablespoons "Chicky Baby Seasoning" (p. 124)
- 1 medium carrot, thinly sliced
- 1 medium stalk of celery, thinly sliced

Last Minute Additions:
- 5 cloves garlic, pressed or minced
- 2 teaspoons balsamic vinegar
- 1 tablespoon tamari, shoyu, or soy sauce
- ½ teaspoon **each:** sea salt and black pepper

1. Place all of the "Into the Big Pot" items into a pressure cooker (or a large pot with a tight-fitting lid). Bring to a boil over high heat.

2. Reduce the heat to low. Simmer for 30 minutes if using a pressure cooker, or 50-60 minutes in a regular pot. The soup is done when the peas have lost all semblance of their former selves and are a smooshy mass of green goodness.

3. Remove the bay leaves and kombu and stir in the remaining additions. At this point, you'll want to whisk the soup well (with a wire whisk) so that the watery top layer and thick pea layer become emulsified.

4. Serve hot or warm. This will last for 7-10 days in the fridge. Upon reheating, you may need to add a little water as this will thicken up substantially with time.

Serves 4-5/GF/Green ❄

> **Tip:** Kombu is an indispensable item when you're talkin' beans. A dried sea vegetable, kombu adds nutrients, brings out flavor, and aids digestibility. Dried kombu is available in most health food stores.

Simply Soothing Fresh Tomato Soup

This soup is best in the summer, but great anytime you can get your mitts on some really ripe, organic tomatoes and fresh, fragrant basil. Ah, sweet soup—the elixir of weight loss, health, and happiness.

- ½ cup **each:** diced celery and diced onion (white or yellow)
- 2 tablespoons olive oil, extra-virgin or regular

- 15 oz. can tomato sauce (with salt)
- 3 medium or 2 large tomatoes (it's crucial to use fresh, ripe tomatoes here)
- ¼ cup (packed) fresh basil leaves
- 1 teaspoon **each:** dried oregano, sea salt, and dried marjoram
- ½ teaspoon dried thyme
- 3 medium cloves garlic, pressed or minced
- ¾ cup nondairy milk, plain and unsweetened
- ¼ teaspoon ground black pepper
- 1 tablespoon **each:** nutritional yeast and agave nectar

1. Set a medium soup pot over medium-high heat. Add the celery and onion and sauté in the oil, stirring often, for 3-5 minutes (or until the onion just begins to brown). Remove from heat.

2. Place the onion-celery mixture in a blender along with all of the remaining ingredients. Blend until as smooth as possible. Which is pretty smooth, when you come to think about it.

3. Place the velvety goodness back into the soup pot and bring to a boil over medium-high heat. Reduce heat to low and simmer for about 10-15 minutes to marry the flavors. Remove from heat and serve. This will keep for up to one week, refrigerated in an airtight container.

Serves 4/GF/SF/Green

Savory Sage and Red Lentil Soup

Although this soup is very low in fat and calories, it's extremely satisfying. So satisfying, in fact, that the mere mention of it makes my lips quiver.

First:
- 1 extra large onion, finely chopped
- 1 tablespoon olive oil

For the Love of Lentils:
- 6 cups water, preferably purified
- 1 cup red lentils, rinsed well and sorted

Savory Seasonings:
- ¼ teaspoon **each:** ground ginger and ground nutmeg
- 1 tablespoon "Chicky Baby Seasoning" (p. 124)
- 1 teaspoon **each:** ground sage and ground thyme
- Fresh ground pepper (I use quite a bit)

Last Additions:
- 1-2 teaspoons sea salt (to taste)
- 4 medium garlic cloves, minced or pressed
- 1 tablespoon fresh lemon juice
- 1 teaspoon tamari, soy sauce, or shoyu
- 1¼ teaspoons balsamic vinegar
- ⅓ cup nondairy milk, plain and unsweetened

1. In a large soup pot set to medium-high heat, sauté the onion in the olive oil. Stir often and cook until the onions are soft and translucent.

2. Add the water and lentils to the soup pot and bring to a boil. Reduce heat to low and add the savory seasonings. Stir well. Simmer for 45 minutes to an hour, or until the lentils have dissolved.

3. Stir in the last additions and serve. Mmmm. This will keep for at least a week refrigerated in an airtight container.

Makes 6 servings/GF/Green ❄

Green Chili-Garlic-Potato Soup

This delicious soup is serious medicine! Green chilies are immune-boosting and extremely high in vitamin C. Plus, the abundance of fresh garlic is the perfect natural antibiotic. Make sure not to overdo it though—green chilies are sublime in moderation, but can upset the tummy if eaten in excess. Trust me.

First:
- 1 cup diced onion
- 1 tablespoon olive oil

Next:
- 4 cups **each:** chopped potatoes (skins on if organic) and water

Last:
- 1 cup roasted, peeled, and chopped mild green chilies (I'm a spicy baby and even I use mild chilies in this dish)
- 4 large cloves garlic, minced or pressed
- 1 teaspoon sea salt
- 2 tablespoons **each:** "Chicky Baby Seasoning" (p. 124) and fresh lime juice

1. In a large soup pot set to medium-high heat, sauté the onion in the oil for about 5 minutes. Add the potatoes and water. Cover and bring to a boil over high heat. Reduce heat to low and simmer, uncovered, until the potatoes are tender (about 20 minutes). Remove from heat, but do not drain off the water.

2. With a potato masher, smash the potatoes thoroughly (while they're still in the pot).

3. Add the green chilies and cook over low heat for an additional 3-5 minutes, stirring often. Remove from heat.

4. Add the remaining ingredients and stir well. Serve hot or warm. Hello, yum!

Serves 4/GF/SF/Green ❉

Ah, green chilies . . .

I buy my green chilies locally every fall when they're roasting at every corner stand. To me, the smell of autumn wouldn't be complete without the aroma of roasted chilies in the air! They freeze very well and are much easier to peel when semi-frozen. Simply run cold water over partially thawed chilies and the peels will slip right off.

However, if you don't have access to freshly roasted chilies, you can either buy fresh green chilies and roast them yourself (in your oven's broiler) or simply buy them pre-packaged. The pre-packaged variety are available in the freezer section of most supermarkets and come chopped, peeled, and roasted—perfect for a fast green chili fix!

Hearty Vegetarian Chili

I had to include this recipe from **Radiant Health, Inner Wealth** as it's a top favorite amongst my weight-loss clients. Plus, it has a great track record as a family-pleaser as it's filling, delicious, and flavorful. If you want an authentic "meaty" texture, you may use the meatless crumbles. However, if you don't mind a slightly unusual twist, substitute the browned tempeh as it's even healthier.

- 2 tablespoons olive oil
- 2 small-medium onions, chopped
- 2 cups vegan burger crumbles or browned tempeh*
- 2 cups liquid vegetarian broth (vegetable or vegetarian "chicken")
- 2 cans (15 oz. each) red kidney or pinto beans, with juice (not drained)
- 2 cans (14.5 oz. each) diced tomatoes, with juice (not drained)
- 6 tablespoons chili powder (a blended chili powder mix, not ground chilies)
- ¼ cup tamari, shoyu, or soy sauce
- 10 (yes, ten) medium cloves garlic, minced or pressed
- 2 tablespoons **each:** organic sugar (or agave nectar) and balsamic vinegar

- 2 teaspoons sea salt (or less if you prefer)

1. Heat the oil in a large soup pot over medium-high heat. Add the onions and burger crumbles (or browned tempeh*) and sauté, stirring often, until the onions begin to soften. If necessary, add some of the broth to prevent sticking.

2. Add everything else (except for the salt) and stir well.

3. Reduce the heat to medium-low and simmer, stirring often, until the mixture is thick and the desired consistency is attained. This should take about 30-45 minutes.

4. Stir in the sea salt and serve. Laugh silently to yourself if your guests begin to comment on the best beef chili they've ever eaten.

Serves 8/GF/Green ❄

*If you wish to use tempeh, first sauté 2 cups of crumbled tempeh in a little oil and tamari for 5-10 minutes (or until lightly browned). Then, add as specified.

Eclectic Entrées
• • • • • • • • • • • •

Here are some of my favorite easy, healthy main dishes that are also yum yum yummy!

Triathlon Tostadas

As the name implies, these yummy tostadas are perfect for endurance, strength, and fitness. And don't let the long list of ingredients fool you—this dish is very easy to make and comes together in under 30 minutes. Triumph!

Un-fried Crunchy Tostadas:
- 6 round corn tortillas, preferably made from sprouted or blue corn
- ½ tablespoon (1½ teaspoons) oil (olive or melted coconut)

Quinoa Layer:
- ⅓ cup dry quinoa, rinsed and drained
- ⅔ cup water
- ¼ teaspoon sea salt

Black Bean Layer:
- 15 oz. can black beans (1¾ cups cooked beans), drained and rinsed
- 1½ tablespoons fresh lime juice
- ½ teaspoon **each:** cumin powder, onion granules, and sea salt
- 3 large cloves garlic, minced or pressed
- ⅛ teaspoon ground cayenne powder

Vivacious Veggies:
- ½ cup **each:** grated carrots and grated (or finely chopped) cabbage
- 3 scallions (green onions), trimmed and finely chopped
- 1 tablespoon fresh lime juice
- 1½ avocados, peeled and chopped (¼ avocado per tostada)

1. Preheat your oven to 375° F. Brush or spray the tortillas lightly on both sides with the oil. Next, lay them out on a cookie sheet in a single layer. Bake for 3-5 minutes, then remove from the oven. Flip each tortilla over and place back in the oven for another 3-5 minutes (or until they are crisp and lightly browned). Be careful not to burn!

2. While your corntillas are transforming into tostada shells, you can perform some other magic. Place the quinoa and water in a small pot with a tight-fitting lid. Bring to a boil over medium-high heat. Reduce the heat to low and simmer until all of the water is absorbed, about 15 minutes. Once done, stir in the ¼ teaspoon of sea salt and set aside.

3. Place all of the "Black Bean Layer" ingredients in a blender or food processor. Blend well until very smooth. Transfer to a small pan and heat over a low flame until warm, stirring occasionally.

4. In a small bowl, toss the carrots, cabbage, and scallions with the lime juice. Set aside.

5. Finally, the finish line! To assemble your healthy masterpieces, place the tostada shells on plates and spread with some of the black bean mixture. Next, sprinkle with quinoa and add the veggies. Finally, garnish with the avocado chunks. You did it! Grab a towel—and don't forget your medal.

Makes 6 tostadas (serves 3-6)/GF/SF/Green/30 Minutes or Under!

Storage Tips: Once cooled, the tostada shells can be stored at room temperature in an airtight container for up to a week. The remaining ingredients can be stored individually, refrigerated in separate airtight containers. Happy noshing!

Baked Chimichanga

This dish is so quick, filling, light, and yummy that I make it several times a week! This recipe is for one person but can easily be multiplied to make more servings.

- 1 sprouted or whole grain tortilla (or gluten-free tortilla)
- ½ cup "Perfect Pinto Beans" (p. 109) or fat-free vegetarian refried beans

Optional Filling Additions:
- One whole green chili, roasted, peeled, and chopped
- ¼ cup brown rice (or "Cilantro-Lime Rice," p. 105)
- ¼ cup grated vegan cheese (such as Daiya)

Frying Fake-Out:
- 1 teaspoon oil (preferably coconut or olive)

Fresh Toppings:
- ½ cup Romaine lettuce, chopped or shredded
- Your favorite organic salsa, to taste
- ¼ cup minced onion (red or green)

Optional: 2 tablespoons "Kid's Choice Guacamole" (p. 100)

1. Preheat your oven to 400° F. Lay the tortilla on a flat surface and place the beans (and optional filling ingredients, if using) in the center. Fold the sides of the tortilla in, then roll the bottom of the tortilla up and over the filling so that your creation resembles, yes, an enclosed burrito.

2. Place on an oven-proof pan. Lightly brush (or spray) the entire wrap with the teaspoon of oil. Bake for 5-10 minutes, or until the bottom has become lightly browned. Turn over and bake for another 5-10 minutes, or until the entire tortilla is nicely browned and crisp. Remove from the oven.

3. Place the chimichanga on a plate and top with the lettuce, salsa, onions, and guacamole (if using). Enjoy!

Serves 1/GF (if using a gluten-free tortilla)/SF/Green
30 Minutes or Under! ❀

Ful Mudhamas

I first tried this dish at a wonderful Mid-Eastern restaurant. Although they used fava beans for authenticity, I've found that pinto beans can ful almost anyone.

- 3 cups (or two 15 oz. cans) cooked and drained fava or pinto beans
- 4 teaspoons extra-virgin olive oil
- 3 tablespoons plus 1 teaspoon fresh lemon juice
- 2 tablespoons (packed) minced fresh cilantro or parsley
- ¾ teaspoon sea salt (use less if your beans contain salt)
- 2 small-medium cloves garlic, minced or pressed

Place all of the ingredients in a large bowl and stir well to combine. Serve at room temperature or cold. This will store refrigerated in an airtight container for several days. This dish is also great served with a side of hummus, toasted whole grain pita wedges, and stuffed grape leaves. Yum!

Serves 4/GF/SF/Green/30 minutes or under!

Garlic Veggie Noodle Bowl, Your Way

To me, this is the perfect guilt-free pasta fix! It's easy, yummy, and quick (especially if you have cooked noodles and pre-cut veggies on hand). Plus, it's a great way to get in your two servings of veggies at mealtime! You'll notice that I've given a range of amounts for the garlic and chili sauce. Personally, I always use the high end of that range for maximum flavor. However, this is **your** noodle bowl (hence, the title). Have fun experimenting and making it just right for you!

- 1 cup cooked noodles (soba, udon, rice, or whole wheat), about 2 oz. dry

- 1 teaspoon toasted sesame oil
- 1 tablespoon tamari, divided
- 1-3 medium cloves garlic, peeled and cut into thin slices
- 2 cups veggies, your choice (You can use just one kind or mix and match.)

- 1-3 cloves garlic, pressed (or minced)
- 1-3 teaspoons Thai spicy chili sauce (I use "Thai Kitchen" brand)
- 1 teaspoon toasted sesame seeds (dry toasted in a skillet until browned)

1. If you haven't cooked your noodles yet, do so now. When they're al dente, drain them well and set aside.

2. In a large skillet or wok set to medium-high heat, add the oil, half of the tamari, the sliced garlic, and your veggies. However, if you're using all quick-cooking veggies (such as bok choy and peapods), you'll want to brown the garlic first before adding them.

3. Stir-fry the veggie-garlic mixture, stirring often, until the garlic is browned and the veggies are crisp-tender.

4. Add the noodles, pressed garlic, chili sauce, and remaining tamari to the veggie mixture and gently stir to combine. Serve in a bowl, topped with the sesame seeds. Now it's time to get your noodle fix—and feel good about it!

Serves 1/GF (with gluten-free noodles)/Green/30 Minutes or Under! ❄

Sexy Saucy Noodles

Why sexy? Well, you'll feel satisfied—yet light—after slurping up a bowl of these tasty noodles. At first glance, they might seem fattening, but they really aren't at all. The high veggie content and use of a fiber-rich pasta (as well as the minimal use of fats) make this dish a weight-loss winner!

- 1 cup of the "Thai Skinny Dipping Sauce" (p. 126)
- 6.4 oz. buckwheat soba noodles (½ of a 12.8 oz. package, or two bundles)
- 1 teaspoon toasted sesame oil

Vivacious Veggies:
- 1 teaspoon toasted sesame oil
- 2 teaspoons tamari
- 2 cups **each:** chopped broccoli and sliced shiitake mushroom caps
- 1 cup frozen, shelled edamame (green soybeans)

Optional Fun:
- 1 tablespoon black sesame seeds, raw or toasted
- ¼ cup spiralized or julienne-cut carrots
- ¼ cup fresh bean sprouts

1. Prepare the sauce according to the directions on p. 126 and set aside.

2. Prepare the soba noodles according to the directions on their package. Soba noodles become tender very quickly, so be careful not to overcook. Drain the noodles and gently toss with the 1 teaspoon of toasted sesame oil. Set aside.

3. Set a skillet or wok over medium-high heat and add the remaining teaspoon of oil and the tamari. Add the broccoli and shiitakes and sauté until the broccoli is crisp-tender and bright green. Add the edamame and cook for up to one more minute, or until the edamame is warmed through. Remove from heat.

4. Gently toss the veggies together with the noodles and one cup of sauce. If desired, top with any or all of the "Optional Fun." This will keep for several days, refrigerated in an airtight container. Enjoy, you sexy thang, you!

Serves 4/Green

In A Hurry? Curry!

Even if you don't have the "Indian Spice Blend" on hand, you can still have this entrée on the table in less than 30 minutes. Although this dish isn't as decadent as most Indian curries, it's still totally satisfying and chock-full of flavor. And nutrients. And fiber. And happiness.

Curry Chapter One:
- 2 teaspoons coconut oil (or non-virgin olive oil)
- 2½ tablespoons "Indian Spice Blend" (p. 125)
- 1 cup low-fat coconut milk

Curry Chapter Two:
- 15 oz. can chickpeas (garbanzo beans), drained and rinsed
- 14.5 oz. can diced tomatoes (with garlic and onions), not drained
- 3 cups chopped cauliflower (or broccoli), cut into bite-sized pieces

Final Chapter of Curry:
- 4 cups baby spinach (pre-washed)
- 4 large cloves garlic, minced or pressed
- 1 teaspoon sea salt

1. If you don't have the "Indian Spice Blend" on hand, please whip up a batch according to the directions on p. 125.

2. In a large skillet or wok set to medium-high heat, melt the coconut oil. Next, add the 2½ tablespoons of "Indian Spice Blend" along with the coconut milk and stir well to combine. Cook, stirring often, for one minute.

3. Add the chickpeas, tomatoes (juices and all), and cauliflower. Stir well and cook over medium-high heat for 10 minutes, or until the cauliflower is tender.

4. Add the spinach and stir well. Once the spinach just starts to wilt, stir in the garlic and salt. As soon as the spinach is wilted (but still bright green in color), remove from heat. Voila! Your dinner is served.

Serves 4/GF/SF/Green/30 Minutes or Under! ❄

Tess's Flavorite Burrito

The medley of spicy, sweet, and tangy flavors makes this a party in your mouth!

- One recipe "Cilantro-Lime Rice" (p. 105)
- One recipe "Mango Habanero Sauce" (p. 127)
- One recipe "Kid's Choice Guacamole" (p. 100)

- 3 cups (two 15 oz. cans) black beans, drained and rinsed
- 1 cup shredded or chopped Romaine lettuce
- 2 medium tomatoes, chopped
- ⅓ cup minced red onion
- 6 whole grain tortillas, preferably sprouted (or gluten-free tortillas)

1. Prepare the rice, sauce, and guacamole and set aside.

2. Prepare all of the remaining ingredients and set aside. If desired, you may wish to add a little sea salt to the beans.

3. Place the tortillas in a dry skillet over medium heat until they're warmed through. Remove from heat and evenly place the fillings in the center of each tortilla. Roll up burrito-style and serve. Enjoy the happiness of loving food that loves you back!

Note: If you have leftovers, they can be stored individually in airtight containers in the refrigerator. They will keep for several days that way.

Makes 6 burritos (serves 6)/GF (if using gluten-free tortillas)/SF/Green

Black-eyed Peas with Kale

This is one of those dishes I could practically live on—it's light, easy to throw together, satisfying, and soooo yummy. This entrée works best with soaked peas, so you may want to plan ahead for maximum goodness.

- 1½ cups dry black-eyed peas, soaked in water overnight (or 8-12 hours)
- ½ cup diced onion
- 3½ cups liquid vegetarian "chicken" broth
- 4 bay leaves
- 4-inch piece of kombu (p. 147)

- 2 cups (packed) kale, preferably lacinato (cut into thin ribbons)
- 6 medium cloves garlic, pressed or minced

- 2 teaspoons **each:** sea salt, nutritional yeast, and olive oil
- ¼ cup fresh lemon juice
- *To Taste (optional):* hot sauce of your choice (habanero, tabasco, etc.)

1. Drain the black-eyed peas to remove the soaking water and then rinse them.

2. Place the beans in a pressure cooker (or regular pot with a tight-fitting lid). Add the onion, broth, bay leaves, and kombu and bring to a boil over high heat. Reduce the heat to low and simmer until the black-eyed peas are tender. This will take about 15 minutes in the pressure cooker (after the top begins to spin) or 45 minutes in a regular pot.

3. Once them beans is finally done, drain off most of the excess liquid. Remove the bay leaves and kombu. Next, stir in the kale and garlic. Cook over medium-high heat for about 5 minutes, stirring often, until the kale is wilted. Remove from heat.

4. Stir in the salt, nutritional yeast, olive oil, and lemon juice. Top with some of the hot sauce (if using) and serve.

Serves 4/GF/SF/Green ❆

Moroccan French Lentils

Yeah, I might be really bad at geography, but don't blame the lentils. This dish is a yummy one-pot wonder, perfect for eating uber-light and healthy in a pinch!

Lovely Lentils:
- 1 cup French lentils (or regular lentils if the French are being evasive)
- ½ cup **each:** orange juice and pomegranate juice
- 2½ cups water
- 4 whole cloves
- 1½ teaspoons **each:** ground cumin and ground cinnamon
- 2 tablespoons agave nectar
- *Optional:* Pinch of saffron

Last Additions:
- 1 cup kale, washed well and cut into thin ribbons
- ¾ teaspoon sea salt

1. Place all of the "Lovely Lentils" items in a pressure cooker (or a large pot with a tight-fitting lid). Stir well, cover, and bring to a boil over high heat. Reduce heat to low and simmer until the lentils are tender (although French lentils remain somewhat firm even when done). This will take about 25 minutes in a pressure cooker, or 45 minutes in a regular pot.

2. Remove from heat and stir in the kale and salt. Cover immediately and let sit until the kale has wilted and become tender, about 5 minutes. Enjoy!

Serves 4-6/GF/SF/Green ❄

Cajun Tofu Wraps

I love this wrap. Love it. Then why don't I marry it, you ask? Well, I did propose—it just never gave me a response. Still waiting, still marinating. Such is life.

Tofu Madness:
- 12 oz. package of firm tofu (water packed), sliced width-wise into 8 cutlets
- 1 tablespoon **each:** fresh lemon juice and tamari
- *To taste:* Cajun spice blend
- 1 teaspoon oil (olive or coconut)

Wrapplings:
- 4 whole grain tortillas, preferably sprouted (or gluten-free tortillas)
- 4 dill pickles, sliced or chopped
- ¼-½ cup low-fat vegan mayonnaise (I use low-fat Vegenaise)
- 1 cup Romaine lettuce, chopped
- Thinly sliced red onions, to taste

1. Gently press the tofu cutlets with paper towels to remove excess water. Place the cutlets in a single layer on a large plate and evenly pour the lemon juice and tamari over them. Allow to marinate for 10 minutes. Turn the tofu over and allow to marinate for another 10 minutes. Sprinkle both sides of the tofu with the Cajun seasoning (to taste, as some like a little and some like it hot—personally, I like to coat each side quite liberally with the seasoning).

2. Set a large skillet over medium heat and add the oil. Place the tofu cutlets in a single layer on the pan and cook until the undersides are browned. Flip over and cook another few minutes until both sides are browned. If you need to do this in batches, so be it. Remove the tofu from heat and set aside.

3. If you like, warm the tortillas in a dry skillet. Place two slabs of tofu in each tortilla and add the remaining items. Wrap up and enjoy the flavor sensation! Rock the nation.

Serves 4/GF (if using a gluten-free tortilla)/Blue

> *Tofu tip:* There's a new product on the market that I recommend trying—it's sprouted tofu (made by Wildwood brand). Sprouting the soybeans makes for an exceptionally fresh, nutritious, and easy to digest food.

Ever So Nice Beans and Rice

This dish is hearty, filling, and flavorful. For an extra kick, feel free to add some chopped cayenne, tabasco, or habanero to the bean mixture (so that it cooks with the beans)—or add a dash of hot sauce at the end. Yum!

- Three 15 oz. cans beans (black-eyed peas or black beans are ideal), with juices (not drained)
- 2 teaspoons **each:** dried oregano, "Chicky Baby Seasoning" (p. 124), and ground cumin
- 2 large bay leaves
- 1 large onion, diced
- 2 fresh tomatoes, diced
- 1 tablespoon balsamic vinegar

Rice:
- 1 cup long grain brown rice
- 2 cups water
- 2 tablespoons "Chicky Baby Seasoning" (p. 124)

Final Freshness:
- 2 tablespoons **each:** fresh lemon juice and minced cilantro
- 5 medium cloves garlic, minced or pressed
- Sea salt, to taste

1. In a large pot, combine the beans, oregano, "Chicky Baby Seasoning," cumin, bay leaves, onion, tomatoes, and balsamic vinegar. Bring to a boil over high heat. Reduce the heat to low and simmer, uncovered, for about 45 minutes. You'll want to stir this every 15 minutes or so while it's cooking.

2. While the beans are doing their deal, rice it up. Place the rice, water, and seasoning in a covered pot and bring to a boil. Reduce heat to low and simmer for about 45 minutes, or until the rice is tender and the water has been absorbed. This should time out quite nicely with the beans.

3. Once the beans are done, stir in the lemon juice, cilantro, garlic, and salt. Serve over the cooked rice. If you like, this can also be garnished with additional cilantro, diced onion, and lemon wedges.

Serves 6/GF/SF/Green ❄

Low-Fat Basil Garlic Linguine

Don't let the title fool you—this dish is more than a calorie saver. It's extremely delicious, flavorful, and satisfying as well! Plus, the uncooked sauce makes it very fresh and a snap to prepare. Enjoy the love.

- 8 oz. whole grain linguine (or whole grain gluten-free pasta if you are gluten intolerant)

Sublime Sauce:
- 1 tablespoon **each:** olive oil and balsamic vinegar
- 15 oz. can crushed tomatoes, lightly drained
- 4-5 medium cloves garlic, pressed or minced
- 2 teaspoons dried oregano
- ¼ cup (packed) fresh basil, cut into thin ribbons
- 1 teaspoon sea salt
- Freshly ground pepper to taste (I use about ½ teaspoon)

1. Begin cooking the linguine according to the directions on the package.

2. While the noodles are cooking, you can place the ingredients for the sauce in a large bowl. You can. . . and you will.

3. When the linguine is al dente, drain and toss with the sauce. Serve immediately. All right!

Serves 4/GF (with substitution)/SF/Blue/30 minutes or under!

Cilantro-Lime Potadas

You'll forgive the silly name for these unusual potato tostadas once you see how pretty they are—and also when you taste the fresh, tangy filling! Serious yum.

- 4 corn tortillas, preferably made from sprouted or blue corn

Thrilling Filling:
- 2 cups chopped potato (one fairly large potato), unpeeled
- ¼ cup finely minced onion, yellow or white
- 2 tablespoons chopped cilantro
- 1 tablespoon olive oil
- 5 teaspoons fresh lime juice
- ½ teaspoon sea salt
- ¼ teaspoon ground turmeric

Garnish:
- 8 kalamata olives, chopped or sliced
- 2 tablespoons **each:** minced cilantro and finely chopped red cabbage
- *Optional:* 4 lime wedges (one lime, quartered)

1. Preheat your oven to 375° F. Spray (or brush) the tortillas lightly on both sides with a little oil and lay out on a cookie sheet in a single layer. Bake for 3-5 minutes, then remove. Flip each tortilla over and bake for another 3-5 minutes (until they're crisp and lightly browned). Be careful not to burn!

2. While the tortillas are in the oven, place the chopped potatoes in a cooking pot and cover completely with water. Bring to a boil over high heat. Reduce heat to low and simmer until the potatoes are tender, about 15 minutes.

3. Drain the potatoes and place back in the pot. Mash with a potato masher. Add the remaining "Thrilling Filling" items to the potatoes. Stir very well to combine.

To serve: Top the tostada shells with the potato filling and sprinkle with the garnishes. For extra tang, squeeze a lime wedge over each tostada. Yummy!

Serves 4/GF/SF/Green/30 Minutes or Under!

> *Tip:* You can also serve the filling as a delicious stand-alone side dish. Think of it as Mexican mashed potatoes with a twist.

Garam Masala Chickpea Curry

Get curried away.

- 1 cup dry chickpeas, soaked in plenty of water for 8-12 hours
- 14.5 oz. can diced tomatoes, not drained
- 1½ cups water
- ½ cup sliced or chopped onions (white or yellow)
- 1 tablespoon garam masala (available in most health food stores)
- ⅛ teaspoon ground cayenne powder (optional)

- 1 tablespoon fresh lime juice
- 1½ cups trimmed green beans (fresh or frozen)
- 1 tablespoon coconut oil
- 1 teaspoon sea salt

1. Drain the chickpeas, then place in a pressure cooker or large pot with a tight-fitting lid. Add the tomatoes, water, onions, garam masala, and cayenne. Bring to a boil over high heat, then reduce heat to low. Simmer until the chickpeas are tender (about 40 minutes in a pressure cooker or 1½ hours in a regular pot).

2. Stir in the lime juice, green beans, oil, and salt. Cook over medium heat for another minute or two, just until the green beans are crisp-tender. Serve plain or alongside brown basmati rice. This will keep for a week or so, refrigerated in an airtight container. Enjoy!

Serves 4/GF/SF/Green ❄

Guilt-Free Desserts

• • • • • • • • • • • • • •

One of the reasons why the Two-Week Wellness Solution is a permanent solution can be found in this chapter. For most of us, feeling deprived doesn't really work long term—and one of the best ways to feel satisfied is to indulge in a seemingly decadent dessert. In this chapter, you'll find you can enjoy everything from rich cheezcake to creamy star bars to gooey cobbler, all minus the guilt. Plus, these delicious desserts come with an added bonus. They'll give your skin a glow and your body a lightness—while still satisfying the kid in you that loves a little sweetness!

Lemon Coconut Vanilla Bean Cheezcake

No, I haven't lost my mind. This really is a weight-loss recipe! How could I possibly think so, you ask? First of all, it uses only raw, real-food ingredients like almonds and cashews. Next, coconut was intentionally chosen as it boosts both immune function and metabolism. These nutrient-dense foods, especially in their raw state, leave you feeling satisfied and nourished—two important things in the long-term weight-loss winners circle. This is a "blue" recipe, so one serving per day still fits in perfectly with the two-week plan. Enjoy!

Crumble Crust:
- 1 cup raw almonds (whole and untoasted)
- ¼ cup (packed) dates, pitted
- 2 tablespoons (packed) raisins
- ⅛ teaspoon sea salt

Fantastically Fresh Filling:
- 1½ cups raw, unsalted cashews
- ¾ cup agave nectar
- ½ cup **each:** fresh lemon juice and coconut butter (see p. 171 for details)
- 1 tablespoon (packed) lemon zest (the zest of two large organic lemons)
- ¼ teaspoon sea salt
- The innards of 1 vanilla bean*

Toptional:
- ½ cup fresh or frozen raspberries
- The zest of one organic lemon
- ⅛ cup finely shredded coconut

1. Place the cashews in plenty of water to cover and let soak for 8-12 hours or overnight. Drain well in a strainer and set aside.

2. *To make the crust*: Place the almonds, dates, raisins, and salt in a food processor. Blend very well, but just until the mixture resembles coarse crumbs and is beginning to stick together. You still want to retain a crumbly consistency, so don't over-blend. Transfer the mixture to a round pie pan and press well with the palms of your hands to form a bottom crust. I usually don't bring the mixture up the sides—it should simply form a nice, thick foundation for the cheezcake topping. Once you've pressed it enough to make a firmly compacted and even

surface, set it aside in the fridge or freezer while you make the filling.

3. *Filling station:* Place the soaked, drained cashews in a clean food processor and blend very well. Add all of the remaining filling ingredients and keep blending. Occasionally, you'll need to scrape down the inside of the food processor with a rubber spatula during this process (while it's off, of course!). Keep blending until very smooth and creamy—it may take a while! Remove and pour/scrape into the pie pan, over the crust. Smooth out the top and place in the freezer for one hour, or until firm (yet not frozen solid).

4. If desired, you can top with any of the following: raspberries, additional lemon zest, and/or finely shredded coconut. Make it purty. This pie will re-freeze very nicely, wrapped in plastic or in an airtight container. Store the remaining portion of the pie (that you don't want to freeze) in the fridge for up to 10 days.

Makes 12 servings/GF/SF/Blue ❄

*To retrieve the vanilla bean innards is very, very simple. I promise. First, make a lengthwise cut down the side of the bean with a sharp knife. Then, open up the pod and scrape out the dark, gooey inside portion using the back of a knife, spoon, or even your fingernail. Place all of the gooey goodness into the mixture.

Coconut butter. . . is not the same as coconut oil. Coconut butter is a divine, raw, whole food that also contains the meat of the coconut. Another way to explain the difference between coconut butter versus coconut oil is to think of the difference in viscosity between peanut butter and peanut oil. Coconut butter can be found in most health food stores or online.

Zingy Grilled Orange-Ginger Grapefruit

When my daughter saw me eating this, she said: "Hmmm. . . that looks like something I'll like when I'm older!" No matter what your age, this is the perfect way to indulge your sweet tooth while still making a healthy choice. Plus, it's the essence of simple, quick, and delicious!

- One grapefruit, cut in half
- 1 tablespoon organic sugar (or agave nectar)
- 2 teaspoons **each:** orange juice and minced crystallized ginger (the ginger should be well packed)
- 1 teaspoon (or slightly less if you prefer) minced orange zest

1. Preheat your oven to broil.

2. Place the grapefruit halves in an upright position in an oven-proof pan or dish. (I use a small glass dish that props the grapefruit up evenly—you want the surface of the grapefruit to be able to retain the juices.)

3. Evenly sprinkle the sugar (or drizzle the agave) over the surface of both grapefruit halves. Sprinkle with the orange juice, ginger, and orange zest.

4. Broil for about 5 minutes (checking often to prevent burning), or until the tops are nicely browned in parts. Remove and enjoy.

Serves 2/GF/SF/Green/30 Minutes or Under!

Cleansing Cucumber Lemonade

Cleansing, unusual, and soooo refreshing! This isn't exactly a traditional dessert, but on a hot summer day it's just the thing to satisfy a sweet tooth. Cucumber, lemon, and lime also work to alkalinize the body—one trick many swear by to help shed weight naturally and gain health (see p. 84 more more on the subject).

- 1 cup **each:** water and peeled, chopped cucumber
- 5 tablespoons fresh lemon juice (the juice of about 2 lemons)
- 4 teaspoons fresh lime juice (the juice of about ½ lime)
- 4 tablespoons agave nectar

1. Place the water and cucumber in a blender. Blend until emulsified.

2. Strain out the pulp using a fine mesh strainer. Discard the pulp (or come up with a fabulous use for it—and e-mail me about it).

3. Blend the strained juice with the remaining ingredients.

4. Serve over ice, garnished with a lime wedge. Say "ahhhh."

Serves 2-4/GF/SF/Blue (if serving 2; Green if serving 4)
30 minutes or under!

Agave nectar is delicious, affordable, and a great replacement for honey. It also boasts a low glycemic index (which means it won't spike your blood sugar as many refined sweeteners tend to do). However, as with all sweeteners it should be used in moderation. Also, be sure to purchase high-quality organic raw agave nectar—found in health food stores.

Tropical Pineapple Napoleons

These are all at once elegant, flavorful, light, and satisfying. Hope you enjoy!

Dynamite Napoleon Layer:
- 5 small sheets of phyllo (or 2½ sheets of larger phyllo),* thawed according to the directions on their package
- 2 teaspoons extra-virgin (or regular) coconut oil, melted

Fruity Booty:
- 15 oz. can pineapple rings (or ten rings of fresh pineapple), drained
- 1 teaspoon extra-virgin (or regular) coconut oil, melted
- 2 teaspoons agave nectar

Glorious Garnish:
- 1 tablespoon **each:** finely shredded coconut and agave nectar

1. Preheat your oven to 400° F. Gently remove the 5 (or 2½)* phyllo sheets from their package and set aside. Securely re-wrap the remaining phyllo in airtight plastic and place back in the fridge for up to 4 weeks.

2. If you have the larger phyllo sheets, cut the whole sheets in half lengthwise. You should now have five phyllo rectangles. Cut each in half to form ten pieces of phyllo. Fold each piece into a 2-inch rectangle. So, unless you're really bad at math (or folding), you should now have ten little phyllo rectangles.

3. Brush a cookie sheet with a little of the 2 teaspoons of coconut oil. Place the phyllo rectangles on the sheet in a single layer and lightly brush with what's left of the 2 teaspoons of oil. Bake until beautifully golden-browned, about 10 minutes (be careful not to burn). Remove and set aside.

4. Set the oven to broil. Lightly oil another baking pan or cookie sheet with ½ teaspoon coconut oil (half of the remaining 1 teaspoon of oil). Place the pineapple rings on the sheet in a single layer and brush with what's left of the oil. Drizzle evenly with the 2 teaspoons of agave nectar. Broil for 5-10 minutes, or until golden-brown on one side. Flip the pieces over and broil for another 5-10 minutes, or until both sides look irresistibly caramelized. Set aside.

5. In a dry pan, toast the grated coconut on low heat until lightly browned. You'll need to shake the pan often (or stir) to prevent burning. Once browned, remove the coconut from the pan immediately. Set aside.

6. To assemble your cute little masterpieces, place one of the phyllo rectangles on a plate. Top with a pineapple ring. On top of that goes another phyllo rectangle. Finish with another pineapple ring. To garnish, top with a sprinkle of toasted coconut and a drizzle of agave nectar. Serve immediately.

Serves 5/SF/Green (if only eating one serving)
30 Minutes or Under!

*If your 1 lb. package of phyllo contains 20 (large) sheets, you will use 2½ of them. If it contains 40 (small) sheets, you will need 5 of them.

Did you know?
Coconut was wrongly accused of being unhealthy for many years. This is because it was linked in studies along with other saturated fats such as lard. Once it was finally isolated and tested on its own, it was acquitted of all charges. For more information on coconut oil, please see p. 58.

Rawberry Star Bars

One of my favorite ways to make guilt-free desserts is to use all raw, living food ingredients. Yet another example that nourishing foods can also be totally satisfying and delicious! These yummy bars have become a favorite in our home as they're so fun and easy to make. If you don't have a star-shaped cookie cutter, you can use any shape you like (or simply cut into squares). Incidentally, these bars are one my favorite ways to get Omega-3s into my daughter's diet with ease—kids absolutely flip for these!

- 1½ cups raw, unsalted cashews
- 2 cups strawberries (or half strawberries, half raspberries), fresh or frozen
- ½ cup **each:** agave nectar and coconut butter
- ¼ cup fresh lemon juice
- 4 teaspoons vanilla extract
- ¼ teaspoon sea salt

1. Place the cashews in plenty of water to cover and let soak for 8-12 hours (or overnight). Drain well in a strainer and set aside.

2. Place the cashews in a food processor and blend very well. Add all of the remaining ingredients and process until smooth. Occasionally, you'll need to scrape down the inside of the food processor with a rubber spatula during this process (while it's off, of course!). Continue to blend until very smooth and creamy. This may take several minutes, so be patient. Remove and pour/scrape into a large lasagna-style pan (9.5 x 13.5-inches). Smooth out the top and place in the freezer for 2 hours, or until mostly firm.

3. Remove from the freezer and cut into stars using a small, star-shaped cookie cutter. If the mixture is too firm to cut, let it thaw for a few minutes first. For the excess portion, you can either shape it into a flat layer, refreeze, and cut into stars again, or simply cut it into randomly shaped chunks. Either way, delish.

4. To store, freeze in an airtight container. To serve, simply remove from the freezer and enjoy immediately (just like you would an ice cream bar).

Makes 20 servings/GF/SF/Blue ❄

Baked Apple with Cinnamon Oat Crumble

This fat-free dessert is the essence of simplicity and ease! Plus, for under five minutes of work, you'll have the comfort of warm cinnamon-apple goodness!

- 1 red apple

Cinnamon Oat Crumble:
- ¼ cup rolled oats
- 2 tablespoons agave nectar
- ½ teaspoon **each:** ground cinnamon and vanilla
- Dash of sea salt (just under ⅛ teaspoon)

1. Preheat the oven to 400° F. Cut the apple in half. With a sharp knife and/or spoon, remove the stem and core from each half of the apple, being careful to leave them intact.

2. Place both apple halves (skin side down) in a baking dish. Cover and bake for 10-15 minutes, or until the apple begins to soften.

3. In a small bowl, combine the oats, agave, cinnamon, vanilla, and salt. Stir well with a spoon and set aside.

4. Remove the apple halves from the oven and uncover. Top each half evenly with the oat mixture and place back in the oven (uncovered). Bake for another 10-15 minutes, or until the topping is lightly browned and the apple is very tender. Serve immediately.

Serves 2/GF (with gluten-free oats)/SF/Green/30 Minutes or Under! ❄

Magical Raspberry Mousse

I don't know why this is magical, but it is. Something to do with the way the tang of the raspberries meets the maple syrup is my best guess. Whatever the reason, I hope you love this light, refreshing dessert as much as I do!

- One 12.3 oz. container of silken tofu, firm or extra firm
- ½ cup pure maple syrup
- 2 cups frozen raspberries (no need to thaw them)
- 1 teaspoon vanilla extract
- ⅛ teaspoon sea salt
- **Optional Garnish:** Fresh raspberries and sprigs of mint

Blend all ingredients in a food processor until completely emulsified. It's just that simple! If desired, top with a few fresh raspberries and a mint leaf.

Serves 6/GF/Blue/30 Minutes or Under!

> *Note:* If you dislike the texture of raspberry seeds, you can do the following:
> Process the raspberries first, then run them through a mesh strainer.
> Finally, process the seedless raspberry mush with the other ingredients.

> *Want to make this extra impressive?*
> Place 2 tablespoons of slivered or sliced almonds in a small skillet.
> Stir in a little agave nectar, cinnamon, and vanilla and cook over low heat, stirring often, until golden-browned. Cool and top each portion of the mousse with 1 teaspoon of the glazed almonds. Yum!

Blackberry Peach Goodness

Oh my. Ooooh my.

Gooey Goodness Filling:
- 10 oz. fresh or frozen blackberries
- 4 cups chopped fresh, ripe peaches
- 3 tablespoons organic sugar
- 1 tablespoon arrowroot
- 2 tablespoons fresh lemon juice

Too Tasty Topping:
- ½ cup rolled oats
- ⅓ cup whole wheat pastry flour
- 3 tablespoons organic sugar
- 1 teaspoon ground cinnamon
- ½ teaspoon ground nutmeg
- ⅛ teaspoon salt
- 3 tablespoons oil (sunflower, non-virgin olive, or melted coconut)

1. Preheat the oven to 375° F. Lightly oil a round pie pan and set aside.

2. Gently combine the filling ingredients in a large bowl. Place them evenly in the pie pan.

3. In a medium bowl, combine the dry topping ingredients (oats, flour, sugar, cinnamon, nutmeg, and salt). Stir very well to combine.

4. Drizzle the oil into the dry topping mixture and stir well until thoroughly combined. Sprinkle evenly over the berry-peach mixture.

5. Bake for about 40 minutes, or until the mixture resembles a gooey fruit nirvana with a golden-brown topping. Cool slightly and serve immediately. Ooh baby!

Serves about 6/SF/Blue ❄

Prenatal Pudding

Thanks to Dr. John and Mary McDougall for sharing their recipe for "Sunshine Tapioca," which inspired this dessert. For some reason I was crazy about this while pregnant many years ago. Crazy. Even my pregnant friends who tried it couldn't get enough! Maybe it's because tapioca is a renowned tummy-soother and the pudding is bursting with fruity-good vitamins. Whatever the reason, you don't have to be pregnant—or a woman—to enjoy this light, citrusy dish.

- 3 tablespoons whole tapioca (not instant)
- 1 cup orange juice (the fresher the better!)
- 20 oz. can pineapple (in its own juices), crushed or tidbits, not drained
- 2 tablespoons fresh lemon juice
- ½ cup tiny orange segments (clementine or mandarin work best)

1. Soak the tapioca in the orange juice for one or two hours.

2. Place the tapioca-orange juice mixture in a medium cooking pot. Add the pineapple (both the fruit and the juice). Cook over medium heat until the mixture comes to a boil. Remove from heat.

3. Stir in the lemon juice and orange segments. Allow to chill in the fridge (in an airtight container) for at least two hours, or until it begins to firm up. Enjoy!

Serves 4/GF/SF/Green

"Green" Packaged Foods

• • • • • • • • • • • • • • • • • •

Just about everyone has times when they're out, about, and ill prepared when hunger strikes! If this is you—and it will be hours before you can go home and whip up a healthy snack—this list can give you some ideas. Of course, you can also just grab an organic apple or banana from the grocery store if need be. But here are some additional ideas for snacks that get the green light (and label). This is by no means a complete list, but it's what I came up with after scouring the shelves of several supermarkets and health food stores.

Note: In addition to giving you ideas for quick convenience foods, I've also listed some of my favorite pastas, breads, and other items that will fit into the two-week plan. However, not all of the items on this list are ones that I've personally tested. I've simply read the labels and found them to be high in ingredient quality. However, I've noted my favorites with an asterisk so you'll know the ones that are pre-tested and loved by me. Happy shopping!

Beverages:

- Blue Sky lemon seltzer (just filtered water and lemon with some fizz)*
- Eden Foods (Edensoy) nondairy milks*
- Guayaki yerba mate ("Unsweetened Mate")
- Honest Tea ("Just Green Tea")
- Living Harvest hemp milk (unsweetened vanilla or unsweetened original)
- Metro Mint bottled waters (peppermint, lemonmint, or spearmint—these are so refreshing!)*
- Millenium GT Dave's Synergy Kombucha (my favorites are grape, strawberry, guava, gingerberry, and passionberry)*
- Pacific Natural Foods almond milk (low-fat original unsweetened)
- Soy Slender unsweetened soy milk (plain or vanilla)
- Steaz organic green tea with lemon (unsweetened)
- Westsoy organic unsweetened soy milk (plain or vanilla)
- Zevia diet soda (sweetened only with natural stevia leaf—try the root beer or cherry and drink ice cold for the best flavor*

Breads and Tortillas:

- Alvarado Street sprouted wheat tortillas and breads*
- Food For Life brown rice tortillas (great for the gluten-free crowd)
- Food For Life Ezekiel 4:9 sprouted products (breads, English muffins, sprouted corn tortillas, sprouted grain tortillas, burger buns, and pitas)*
- French Meadow "Fat Flush" tortillas
- Manna Organics manna breads (millet-rice, fruit and nut, and cinnamon-date)
- Rudi's "Multigrain Wraps"
- Rudi's "7 Grain with Flax Wraps"

Breakfast Cereals:

- Barbara's "Grain Shop"
- Cascadian Farms "Hearty Morning Fiber"*
- Food For Life Ezekiel 4:9 ("Original" or "Golden Flax")*
- Kashi "Autumn Wheat"*
- Kashi "Island Vanilla"*
- Nature's Path "Heritage High Fiber" (flakes)*
- Nature's Path "Organic Flax Plus" ("Pumpkin Raisin Crunch")
- Nature's Path "Organic Smart Bran"*

Breakfast Items (see also frozen foods):

- Arrowhead Mills instant oatmeal (original plain)
- Arrowhead Mills nondairy pancake and waffle mixes (buckwheat or kamut)
- Arrowhead Mills "Organic Rice and Shine Hot Cereal"
- Arrowhead Mills organic yellow corn grits
- Bob's creamy rice hot cereal ("Brown Rice Farina")
- Bob's organic high-fiber oat bran hot cereal
- Nature's Path organic instant hot oatmeal ("Flax Plus," "Optimum," "Multigrain Raisin Spice," "Apple Cinnamon," "Maple Nut," or the variety pack)

Frozen Foods:

- Amy's black bean burrito (nondairy)*
- Amy's brown rice and bean burrito (nondairy)*

- Amy's brown rice and vegetables bowl
- Amy's brown rice bowl ("Black-eyed Peas and Veggies")
- Amy's multigrain hot cereal bowl
- Amy's "Shepherd's Pie"*
- Amy's steel cut oats bowl
- Amy's tamales ("Roasted Vegetables" or "Verde Black Bean")*
- Amy's "Teriyaki Bowl"
- Amy's "Veggie Loaf Meal"*
- Edamame (any brand as long as it's organic—I buy the shelled version)*
- Rice Expressions (organic rice pilaf and organic brown rice)
- Sambazon acai berry puree (great in smoothies!)*
- Sunshine Burgers (southwest, barbecue, garden herb, or breakfast)

Pastas:

- Ancient Harvest Organic Supergrain pastas (a personal favorite—this yummy corn-quinoa pasta comes in lots of varieties including linguine, garden pagodas, veggie curls, shells, elbows, and spaghetti)*
- Bionaturae 100% whole wheat pastas*
- Buckwheat soba noodles (any organic brand such as Koyo)*
- Eden noodles (any whole grain variety such as udon)
- Koyo organic ramen noodles (I toss lots of veggies in with them for a five minute meal when I need something fast!)*
- Tinkyada organic brown rice pastas

Pasta Sauces:

- Muir Glen ("Tomato Basil," "Fire Roasted Tomato," "Garlic Roasted Garlic," and "Garden Vegetable")*

Refrigerated Items:

- Lightlife "Fakin' Bacon" (smoky tempeh strips)*
- Nancy's plain soy yogurt*
- Rejuvenative Foods ("Zing Salad," "Garden Kim-Chi," "Spicy Kim-Chi," and "Raw Sauerkraut")
- Turtle Island marinated tempeh ("Coconut Curry" or "Sesame Garlic")
- Turtle Island tempeh (spicy veggie, soy, or 5-grain)
- West Soy tempeh

Salad Dressings:

- Newman's Organic Light Balsamic*
- Newman's Organic Low-Fat Asian

Seasonings:

- Simply Organic fajita seasoning (great with sliced tempeh or tofu)*
- Simply Organic seasoned salt*
- Simply Organic sloppy joe mix (use with crumbled tempeh)

Snacks:

- Amazing Grains organic green super food bar ("Berry Whole Food Energy Bar" or "Whole Food Energy Bar")
- Bearitos "Lite" popcorn
- Clif "C" bars (try the blueberry*)
- Foods Alive organic flax crackers ("Italian Zest," "Mustard," "Onion-Garlic,"* "BBQ," "Hemp," "Original," and "Maple and Cinnamon")
- Freeland Foods Go Raw flax bars ("Banana 'Bread'" or "Real Live")
- Freeland Foods Go Raw "Flax Snax" (simple, sunflower, or spicy)
- Freeland Foods Go Raw "Spirulena Energy Bar"
- Freeland Foods Go Raw "Super Chips" (spirulena* or pumpkin)
- Grainaissance mochi ("Super Seed," "Sesame-Garlic," "Original," "Cashew-Date," and "Raisin and Cinnamon")*
- Kaia Foods Buckwheat Crunchies raw granola ("Dates and Spices")
- Kaia Foods raw buckwheat granola ("Raisin Cinnamon")
- Koyo organic brown rice chips*
- Lundberg organic brown rice cakes (plain, tamari, seaweed, or wild rice)*
- Mary's Gone Crackers "Sticks and Twigs" (try the sea salt variety)*
- Mary's Gone Crackers whole grain crackers (original, herb, onion, or black pepper)*
- Nutiva Hempseed Bar, original
- Organic ReBar ("Organic Fruit and Veggie Bar")
- Oskri Quinoa Bar
- Raw Revolution Organic Life Food Bar ("Spirulena and Cashew" or "Tropical Mango")
- Real Foods corn thins*
- Sound Sea Vegetables ("Spicy Nori Strips"—my daughter's addiction)*

- Two Moms In the Raw granola (blueberry, gluten-free blueberry, cranberry, gojiberry, or raisin)*
- Two Moms In the Raw sea crackers ("Pesto" or "Garden-Herb")

Soups and Broths:

- Amy's black bean vegetable (low-fat)
- Amy's chunky vegetable (fat-free)
- Amy's split pea (low-fat)
- Amy's vegetable barley (low-fat)
- Imagine acorn squash and mango (nondairy)
- Imagine corn chipotle bisque (nondairy)
- Imagine creamy sweet pea (nondairy)
- Imagine creamy tomato (nondairy)*
- Imagine "No Chicken Broth"
- Imagine vegetable broth

*Items that are marked with an asterisk are those that I have personally tested and enjoyed. Those without an asterisk might be just as yummy, but I haven't tried them—I have only found their ingredients to be high in quality and worthy of the "green" label.

After the Plan: Radiant Health for Life!

• •

First things first—congratulations! I'm so happy that you've made it through the two weeks and I'm giving you a virtual hug and pat on the back right now (did you feel that?). I hope you've gained loads of health benefits and wisdom from following the two-week plan and are now feeling fantastic. And just think, this is only the beginning! Just by completing the two-week program, you have set the tone for increased wellness on all levels—for the rest of your life. You now know that you are in control of your health and wellness. You also know that you can look and feel your best simply by choosing to love foods that love you back. Yay!

Before we move on, however, I'd like to encourage you to take a few moments to reflect. Start by writing down in a journal or notebook what you've gained from following this program. How much weight did you lose? What kinds of health benefits did you experience? Did you enjoy a heightened level of inner wellness? In my experience, journaling this information can be very useful (especially if you ever get off track) as it will remind you that you can always choose optimum wellness just by altering your habits.

So, are you ready to move forward and experience even more abundant wellness? Great! This chapter will help you choose a customized lifestyle that works for you. I've outlined three basic plans that are sure to keep you thriving and at your healthiest weight. You can even pick and choose aspects from them to customize your own personal plan. Whatever works! Because this is all about what works for you and what will end the cycle of "dieting" forever. This is about loving your lifestyle, feeling satisfied, and enjoying your maximum state of wellness on all levels—for life. You deserve it!

Option One: "The Two-Week Wellness Solution for Life"

"I could keep on doing the two-week plan forever!"

I hear this from many participants after they complete the two-week program. If you're like them, this option is for you. It allows for a little more flexibility but honors the basic principles of the two-week plan. Of course, if you do wish to continue on with the Two-Week Wellness Solution just as it's outlined on pages 15-16, it's perfectly safe. Just make sure to eat enough (aim for level three of the hunger and fullness gauge) and always listen to your body.

Morning: Lemon Water, optional "Green Radiance," (p. 86), and fresh fruit (or a smoothie)

Mid-Morning: Healthy snack ("green")

Lunch: Two servings of veggies/"green" foods

3 p.m.: Two servings of veggies/"green" foods

Dinner: Two servings of veggies/a bean-based "green" dish

- Up to three dinners weekly may include starchy foods such as rice, potatoes, whole grain pasta, or quinoa.
- Up to one serving of a "blue" food daily is fine.
- Each week, you may eat up to two servings of a "purple" food (see note below) or three additional "blue" foods.
- Never eat past level three of the hunger and fullness gauge (located on p. 12)

> *Note:* "Purple" signifies plant-based foods that are higher in simple sugars and/or fats. An example would be "Chocolate Decadence Cake" (from my book ***Radiant Health, Inner Wealth***). They are still acceptable ***in moderation*** as they don't contain hydrogenated oils, animal products, artificial ingredients, etc.

Option Two: "Radiant Health and Wellness for Life"

"I loved the two-week plan but I want more flexibility. Plus, I don't know if I can keep eating six cups of vegetables daily."

Sound familiar? Then this option may be just your ticket.

Morning: Lemon Water, optional "Green Radiance," (p. 86), and fresh fruit (or a smoothie)

Mid-Morning: Snack ("green")

Lunch: Two servings of veggies/"green" foods

Afternoon Snack: "green" or "blue" choices

Dinner: Two servings of veggies/"green" foods

- You may have up to two servings of a "blue" food daily.
- Each week, you may have up to two servings of a "purple" food.
- Never eat past level three of the hunger and fullness gauge (located on p. 12)

Option Three: "G.L.E.E. For Life"

"In the long run, I would do better without a structured guideline. I am able to stay in balance and make healthy choices by listening to my body."

Is this you? Great! You'll enjoy the freedom and effectiveness of the G.L.E.E. principles. And although this option is much less structured, you will still lose weight (and/or maintain your healthiest weight) if you consciously apply each aspect.

Good stuff—emphasize it

This "G" principle encourages you to emphasize the good things—vitalizing foods that will nourish you and keep you thriving. These include lots of fresh vegetables (the ideal being at least six servings daily), fruits, beans, and whole grains. Additionally, you'll want to continue eating mainly "green" foods while allowing "blue" and "purple" foods in moderation. However, there are no rules here—just let your own inner wisdom be your guide. Simply by putting your focus on the "good stuff," you'll automatically eat less (if any) of the not-so-good stuff.

Listen

Listening to your own inner wisdom is one of the best habits you can cultivate—it will positively affect everything in your life and give you insight and confidence. By developing the habit of truly listening to your body, you will become your own best nutritionist. Your body will always tell you what it needs for optimum health. Of course, this does take practice—but it's worth it!

By listening to your body, you will also become attuned to what your true cravings are. Remember, true cravings represent what your body really needs, while false cravings represent toxins your body is holding onto (or mental cravings for foods you've had attachments to in the past). By developing the habit of listening, you will always know what your true cravings are and how to satisfy them healthfully and enjoyably.

Eat less

This one is simple—it only takes awareness and commitment. In a nutshell, the "E" principle just means that you're not eating past level three of the hunger and fullness gauge (p. 12). In other words, you are always mindful to eat only until you're *just* satisfied. Merely this simple act of not overeating will do wonders to keep you at your healthiest weight (and in a state of radiant health and wellness) for life.

Exercise

Shake it up! Regular exercise will help keep your metabolism up, your mood elevated, and your heart healthy. I recommend creating an exercise routine that is just right for you—one that you can enjoy sticking with and that motivates you. I also recommend variety when it comes to exercise. For best results overall, try to fit in some strength training, stretching, and cardiovascular exercise each week. Develop a program that is doable and fun for you and that helps you meet your goals. As always, you are worth it!

Final Thoughts

I hope that you are now feeling empowered and excited about the next part of your journey. At this point, you've completed the two-week plan, journaled about your experiences, and decided on the best approach for your long-term health and success. With any luck, you've begun to actually prefer health-supporting foods and are enjoying your new lifestyle tremendously.

I'd like to leave you with two simple reminders. First, always remember your potential. The human body was designed to function in a state of optimal health and wellness—it is capable of far more than we realize. You are meant to thrive, enjoy life, and live in a state of health and harmony. Claim that!

Second, I'd like to remind you that you don't always have to be perfect. As I stated on p. 19, my most successful clients and participants weren't always the most "perfect" ones. They were simply determined to succeed, and they always got back on track no matter how many times they "fell off the wagon."

So, my final suggestion is to be kind and gentle with yourself—while at the same time honoring your vast potential for healthy change. You can do anything you set your mind to! And what could be more important than your own health and wellness? For the truth is that the healthier and happier you allow yourself to be, the more you will be able to share with others. Mahatma Gandhi once said: "Be the change you wish to see in the world." So, let's all be that change and shine a light of health and joy for others. Namaste.

Recommendations and Resources

· ·

Some of my favorite prepared Foods:

- *GT Synergy kombucha:* Addictively delicious and revitalizing? Sign me up! My favorites are the grape, strawberry, guava, and passionberry. One kombucha daily would be considered "green."

- *Earth Café:* Delicious raw vegan cheesecakes that are made solely from good ingredients! My favorites are the lemon, raspberry, and strawberry. One slice of any of their cheesecakes would be considered "blue." www.earthcafetogo.com

- *Daiya vegan cheese*: A revolution for cheezy vegans like me! I order mine from Pangea (www.veganstore.com). This would be considered "blue."

- *Nancy's soy yogurt:* The only vegan yogurt I adore—so fresh and vitalizing! I buy the plain quart-sized yogurts by the case. One ½ cup serving of this would be "green."

For more acceptable packaged items, please refer to "'Green' Packaged Foods" on pages 181-185.

Books:

- *Radiant Health, Inner Wealth:* This is the 2nd edition of my complete guide to wellness, including over 240 color-coded recipes that will keep you eating well for a very long time! www.RadiantHealth-InnerWealth.com

- *The New Whole Foods Encyclopedia* by Rebecca Wood: This is my whole foods "bible" as it contains everything you could ever want to know about plant-based foods. www.amazon.com

- *Local Wild Life* by Katrina Blair: This book is a treasure of delicious living foods, written with love. www.TurtleLakeRefuge.org

- *The Thrive Diet* by Brendan Brazier: Inspired recipes and expert advice from a vegan ironman triathlete. www.amazon.com

- *Vegan Bodybuilding and Fitness* by Robert Cheeke: An excellent guide for beginners or advanced athletes. Robert gives you indispensable information on achieving top performance, using the vegan edge. www.veganbodybuildingbook.com

- *Happy Herbivore* by Lindsay S. Nixon: Lindsay's blog (www.HappyHerbivore.com) is a great resource for low-fat, healthy vegan recipes. Also, look for her cookbook, *The Happy Herbivore Cookbook*, due out in January 2011.

Kitchen Resources:

- *Pampered Chef garlic press:* You don't even have to peel the cloves—so convenient!

- *Excalibur food dehydrator:* The best food dehydrator I know of. I have the big daddy (nine tray model) and love it!

- *SoyaPower soymilk maker:* A great investment—ours paid for itself in about four months.

- *Cuisinart food processors:* I've always had great luck with this brand of food processors.

- *Benriner spiralizer:* Fun for making angelhair-like strands of carrots, beets, potatoes, or zucchini. A great tool for raw foods (and kid-friendly veggies).

- *Deni yogurt maker:* A great way to ensure high quality, fresh vegan yogurt. Easy to use and inexpensive.

Notes

• • • •

[1] Dr. Mehmet Oz "Dr. Oz's Ultimate Aging Checklist" from the show *Dr. Oz Reveals the Ultimate Checklist for Great Aging.* Originally aired on February 5, 2008. www.oprah.com

[2] Dr. John McDougall, "Fish is Not a Health Food" from *The McDougall Newsletter* (February 2003)

[3] Dr. John McDougall, *The McDougall Plan* (page 3)

[4] Dr. John McDougall, *The McDougall Plan* (page 102)

[5] Dr. John McDougall, "Protein Overload" from *The McDougall Newsletter* (January 2004)

[6] Rebecca Wood, *The New Whole Foods Encyclopedia* (page 93)

[7] Richard Weinstein, DC (quote taken on 4/10/2010 from From Dr. Anca Martalog's website, www.askdoctoranca.com on the page www.askdoctoranca.com/30ways)

[8] Firman E. Baer Report, Rutgers University Study

[9] Environmental Working Group Study (Washington D.C.) www.erg.org

[10] Jesse Ziff Cool (*Your Organic Kitchen*) and the Environmental Working Group Study (Washington D.C.) www.erg.org

[11] Brendan Brazier, *Thrive: The Vegan Nutrition Guide to Optimal Performance in Sports and Life* (page 48)

Index

. . . .

A

B

F

G

H

I

M

Q

R

S

May your life be full of joy, overflowing health, peace, and love.
May you also never forget who you truly are—a being with unlimited
potential who is always capable of beautiful transformation.

. . . And don't forget to have fun on your journey!

www.RadiantHealth-InnerWealth.com